Iris Chi, DSW
Kalyani K. Mehta, PhD
Anna L. Howe, PhD
Editors

Long-Term Care in the 21st Century: Perspectives from Around the Asia-Pacific Rim

Long-Term Care in the 21st Century: Perspectives from Around the Asia-Pacific Rim has been co-published simultaneously as *Journal of Aging & Social Policy*, Volume 13, Numbers 2/3 2001.

Pre-publication REVIEWS, COMMENTARIES, EVALUATIONS . . .

"**W**ELL RESEARCHED AND RELEVANT. . . . I especially appreciate this book as we in the World Health Organization continue our efforts to prepare sound long-term care policy advice to our Member States. The thoughtful analysis presented in the manuscript–especially the chapters describing new efforts in long-term care policy development in countries where family structure and social context are rapidly changing–is most informative."

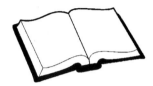

Dr. Miriam J. Hirschfeld, CCL
Director
Noncommunicable Diseases and Mental Health
World Health Organization

More Pre-publication
REVIEWS, COMMENTARIES, EVALUATIONS . . .

"**A**N IMPORTANT STUDY. . . .
Provides a unique account of
long-term care from the perspectives
of both academic policy experts and
those directly involved in the policy
and service development process.
REQUIRED READING for all students,
policy makers, and practitioners in the
field of long-term care and, more
generally, for students of gerontology and geriatrics."

Alan Walker, DLitt
Professor of Social Policy
University of Sheffield
United Kingdom

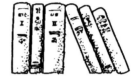

The Haworth Press, Inc.

Long-Term Care in the 21st Century: Perspectives from Around the Asia-Pacific Rim

Long-Term Care in the 21st Century: Perspectives from Around the Asia-Pacific Rim has been co-published simultaneously as *Journal of Aging & Social Policy*, Volume 13, Numbers 2/3 2001.

The *Journal of Aging & Social Policy* Monographic "Separates"

Below is a list of " separates," which in serials librarianship means a special issue simultaneously published as a special journal issue or double-issue *and* as a "separate" hardbound monograph. (This is a format which we also call a "DocuSerial.")

"Separates" are published because specialized libraries or professionals may wish to purchase a specific thematic issue by itself in a format which can be separately cataloged and shelved, as opposed to purchasing the journal on an on-going basis. Faculty members may also more easily consider a "separate" for classroom adoption.

"Separates" are carefully classified separately with the major book jobbers so that the journal tie-in can be noted on new book order slips to avoid duplicate purchasing.

You may wish to visit Haworth's Website at . . .

http://www.HaworthPress.com

. . . to search our online catalog for complete tables of contents of these separates and related publications.

You may also call 1-800-HAWORTH (outside US/Canada: 607-722-5857), or Fax 1-800-895-0582 (outside US/Canada: 607-771-0012), or e-mail at:

getinfo@haworthpressinc.com

Long-Term Care in the 21st Century: Perspectives from Around the Asia-Pacific Rim, edited by Iris Chi, DSW, Kalyani K. Mehta, PhD, and Anna L. Howe, PhD (Vol. 13, No. 2/3, 2001). *Discusses policies and programs for long-term care in the United States, Canada, Japan, Australia, Singapore, Hong Kong, and Taiwan,*

Advancing Aging Policy as the 21st Century Begins, edited by Francis G. Caro, PhD, Robert Morris, DSW, and Jill Norton (Vol. 11, No. 2/3, 2000). *"AN IDEAL TEXTBOOK for any graduate-level course on the aging population. Stands out among existing books on social problems and policies of the aging society. SUCCINCT AND TO THE POINT. A must-read for students, researchers, policy advocates, and policymakers." (Namkee G. Choi, PhD, Professor, Portland State University, Oregon)*

Public Policy and the Old Age Revolution in Japan, edited by Scott A. Bass, PhD, Robert Morris, DSW, and Masato Oka, MSc (Vol. 8, No. 2/3, 1996). *"Anyone seriously interested in the 21st Century and exploring means of adaptation to the revolution in longevity should read this book." (Robert N. Butler, MD, Director, International Longevity Center, The Mount Sinai Medical Center, New York)*

From Nursing Homes to Home Care, edited by Marie E. Cowart, DrPH, and Jill Quadagno, PhD (Vol. 7, No. 3/4, 1996). *"A compendium of research and policy information related to long-term care services, aging, and disability. Contributors address topics encompassing the risk of disability, access to and need for long-term care, and planning for a future long-term care policy." (Family Caregiver Alliance)*

International Perspectives on State and Family Support for the Elderly, edited by Scott A. Bass, PhD, and Robert Morris, DSW (Vol. 5, No. 1/2, 1993). *"The cross-cultural perspectives of the volume and the questions asked about what services are really needed and by whom they should be provided will be useful to the authors' intended audience in gerontological policymaking." (Academic Library Book Review)*

Long-Term Care in the 21st Century: Perspectives from Around the Asia-Pacific Rim

Iris Chi, DSW
Kalyani K. Mehta, PhD
Anna L. Howe, PhD
Editors

Long-Term Care in the 21st Century: Perspectives from Around the Asia-Pacific Rim has been co-published simultaneously as *Journal of Aging & Social Policy*, Volume 13, Numbers 2/3 2001.

The Haworth Press, Inc.
New York • London • Oxford

Long-Term Care in the 21st Century: Perspectives from Around the Asia-Pacific Rim has been co-published simultaneously as *Journal of Aging & Social Policy*™, Volume 13, Numbers 2/3 2001.

The Haworth Press, 10 Alice Street, Binghamton, NY 13904-1580 USA

Cover design by Thomas J. Mayshock Jr.

Library of Congress Cataloging-in-Publication Data

Long-Term Care in the 21st Century: Perspectives from Around the Asia-Pacific Rim / Iris Chi, Kalyani K. Mehta, and Anna L. Howe, editors.
     p. cm.
"Co-published simultaneously as Journal of aging & social policy, volume 13, numbers 2/3 2001."
Includes bibliographical references and index.
ISBN 0-7890-1932-9 (hard : alk. paper) – ISBN 0-7890-1933-7 (pbk: alk. paper)
1. Aged--Long-term care--Pacific Area.
     [DNLM: 1. Long-Term Care. 2. Health Services for the Aged. WX 162 L8485 2002]
I. Chi, Iris. II. Mehta, Kalyani. III. Howe, Anna L. (Anna Louise), 1945- IV. Journal of aging & social policy.
RC954.6.P16 L66 2002
362.1'6'091823--dc21

                                 2002003160

Indexing, Abstracting & Website/Internet Coverage

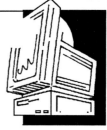

This section provides you with a list of major indexing & abstracting services. That is to say, each service began covering this periodical during the year noted in the right column. Most Websites which are listed below have indicated that they will either post, disseminate, compile, archive, cite or alert their own Website users with research-based content from this work. (This list is as current as the copyright date of this publication.)

Abstracting, Website/Indexing Coverage . . . . Year When Coverage Began

- *Abstracts in Anthropology* 1991

- *Abstracts in Social Gerontology: Current Literature on Aging* 1991

- *Academic Abstracts/CD-ROM* 1994

- *Academic Search Elite (EBSCO)* 1995

- *AgeInfo CD-ROM* 1995

- *AgeLine Database* 1993

- *Biology Digest (in print & online)* 1990

- *Cambridge Scientific Abstracts <www.csa.com>* 1992

- *caredata CD: The social and community care database*
  <www.scie.org.uk> 1996

- *CINAHL (Cumulative Index to Nursing & Allied*
  Health Literature) <www.cinahl.com> 1996

- *CNPIEC Reference Guide: Chinese National Directory*
  of Foreign Periodicals 1995

(continued)

(continued)

*Special Bibliographic Notes related to special journal issues
(separates) and indexing/abstracting:*

- indexing/abstracting services in this list will also cover material in any "separate" that is co-published simultaneously with Haworth's special thematic journal issue or DocuSerial. Indexing/abstracting usually covers material at the article/chapter level.
- monographic co-editions are intended for either non-subscribers or libraries which intend to purchase a second copy for their circulating collections.
- monographic co-editions are reported to all jobbers/wholesalers/approval plans. The source journal is listed as the "series" to assist the prevention of duplicate purchasing in the same manner utilized for books-in-series.
- to facilitate user/access services all indexing/abstracting services are encouraged to utilize the co-indexing entry note indicated at the bottom of the first page of each article/chapter/contribution.
- this is intended to assist a library user of any reference tool (whether print, electronic, online, or CD-ROM) to locate the monographic version if the library has purchased this version but not a subscription to the source journal.
- individual articles/chapters in any Haworth publication are also available through the Haworth Document Delivery Service (HDDS).

Long-Term Care in the 21st Century: Perspectives from Around the Asia-Pacific Rim

CONTENTS

ABOUT THE EDITORS

Iris Chi, DSW, received her Bachelor of Social Science at the Chinese University of Hong Kong in 1978 and obtained her Doctorate in Social Welfare from the University of California, Los Angeles, in 1985. Since 1998, she has held the position of Professor and Director of the Centre on Ageing at the University of Hong Kong. She has published over 50 articles in regional and international refereed journals; other publications include 14 edited books and monographs and 12 book chapters. She has been an invited keynote speaker at many international and regional conferences and has been appointed to policy and academic consultant positions, including membership in the Elderly Commission of the Hong Kong Special Administrative Region, special advisor on aging to the WHO and the UN, advisory board member of the National U.S. Academy of Certified Care Managers, associate fellow of interRAI, and advisor to the International Association of Gerontology Asia-Oceania Region. She is a member of the editorial board of international journals, and has held positions as an honorary professor and research fellow of international research centers on aging, including the University of Victoria, BC, Canada.

Kalyani K. Mehta, PhD, is Associate Professor in the Department of Social Work and Psychology, National University of Singapore. She has done research on elderly services and policies for the past 10 years and has published articles in international and regional journals and presented conference papers in the United States, China, Australia, and South East Asia. As a member of the National Committee on the Aged as well as a consultant to the United Nations Economic and Social Commission for Asia and the Pacific (ESCAP), Dr. Mehta has recommended policies and services for the improved quality of life of older persons. Her edited volume, *Untapped Resources: Women in Aging Societies Across Asia,* published in 1997, added greatly to the literature on the status and roles of older women in aging societies. Her research interests include family caregiving, religion and aging, widowhood, remarriage, and cross-cultural patterns of aging.

Anna L. Howe, PhD, was President of the Australian Association of Gerontology from 1997 to 2000, and she has held academic research and teaching positions in gerontology at the National Ageing Research Institute (1997-98) and its predecessor, the National Research Institute for Gerontology and Geriatric Medicine (1979-87), affiliated with Melbourne University, and at La Trobe University (1987-89 and 1994-96). From 1989-1993, Dr. Howe was Director of the Commonwealth Office for the Aged and also Principal Policy Advisor to the Mid-Term Review of the Aged Care Reform Strategy. She was also a member of the Board of the Australian Institute of Health and Welfare from 1994 to 1998. Internationally, she has carried out consultancies with the OECD and WHO; most recently, she has been a member of the UN Expert Panel on Research and Policy, convened for the International Year of Older Persons, and she has lead a project on aging policy development in China, carried out under the China Capacity Building Program supported by the Australian federal government agency AusAid.

Introduction

This volume is the outcome of a Workshop organized by the Center on Aging at the University of Hong Kong and jointly sponsored by the Elderly Commission of the Hong Kong Government, held in January 2000. The purpose of the Workshop was to canvas recent developments in long-term care for the elderly in seven countries around the Pacific Rim and to assess prospects on the threshold of the 21st Century.

The significance of capturing these perspectives at this particular point in time derives from the rapid pace of change that aged care systems are undergoing in these countries, not so much because of rapid demographic change, which has been recognized for some years now, but more importantly because of social, economic, and political factors that have seen aged care move on to the policy agendas of national governments. Developments in each country are also being influenced by initiatives in the others, and a central aim of the Workshop was to promote comparative analysis to give a better appreciation of the potential for, and limits to, transfers in policy and service delivery. These exchanges are not simply a matter of Japan, Hong Kong, Singapore, and Taiwan taking account of past developments in countries where long-term care systems have been longer established; rather, they further provide opportunities for the United States, Canada, and Australia to revise their own systems in the light of innovations that are coming about as newer systems take shape. The eventual shape that the aged care system takes in each country will depend on the success of the approaches now being implemented. In years to come, it will be important to be able to look back over the current transition period.

Recognizing that policies and programs for long-term care in these countries are at very different stages of development and that each has a different system of government and service delivery, two participants were invited from each country, one to address policy and financing issues and the other to focus

[Haworth co-indexing entry note]: "Introduction." Chi, Iris, Kalyani K. Mehta, and Anna L. Howe. Co-published simultaneously in *Journal of Aging & Social Policy* (The Haworth Press, Inc.) Vol. 13, No. 2/3, 2001, pp. 1-4; and: *Long-Term Care in the 21st Century: Perspectives from Around the Asia-Pacific Rim* (ed: Iris Chi, Kalyani K. Mehta, and Anna L. Howe) The Haworth Press, Inc., 2001, pp. 1-4. Single or multiple copies of this article are available for a fee from The Haworth Document Delivery Service [1-800-HAWORTH, 9:00 a.m. - 5:00 p.m. (EST). E-mail address: getinfo@haworthpressinc.com].

on the organization and delivery of long-term care. A deliberate effort was made to select individuals who had participated directly in policymaking and service development in each country, as well as having academic research and teaching experience. In the case of Hong Kong, for example, Professor Iris Chi is an academic in social work and social policy, and Dr. Edward Leung is a consultant geriatrician practicing in a multidisciplinary team in a not-for-profit hospital and President of the Hong Kong Gerontology Association. Both have served on a number of government advisory bodies and are active in policy debates. Profiles of all contributors are included with their respective articles.

To provide consistency in coverage across all the national systems, a set of themes was identified as a guide for the pairs of papers. The scope of long-term care was first defined as a set of health, personal care, and social services delivered over a sustained period of time to older persons who are medically stable but who have functional disabilities that render them incapable of fully independent self-care, and who thus need multiple services to assist them to live independently in the community, often with support from family members.

Contributors were then asked to address a set of key issues that would assist in gaining a comparative perspective, but at the same time highlight the particular features of long-term care systems in each country that affected the potential for exchange among countries. The discussions of policy and financing set the context for the accounts of service delivery. They begin with reviews of the principles, philosophies, and values that underpin approaches to long-term care; they outline current policy objectives, legislation, and the role of government in developing long-term care; and they then turn to financing arrangements, giving attention to measures adopted to promote budget efficiency and efficacy in resource allocation, and to the relative roles of direct public funding, insurance-based funding, and user co-payments.

The themes for the papers on the organization and delivery of long-term care were first concerned with planning and implementation–service program infrastructure, administration and coordination, selection of service providers and quality management systems–followed by discussion of the "who, what, and when of service delivery," client eligibility and range of services covered, assessment and classification of clients, approaches to case management, and expected outcomes. Within these common frameworks, there is considerable variation in the emphasis given to some of these themes rather than others in the papers from various countries. This variation reflects the differences among the countries in the stage of development of policies and delivery systems; it also enables a focus on the issues identified as priorities as each country entered the 21st century.

The decision on the order in which the countries should follow each other took account not only of the level of aging in each country, but also of the dynamics of policy and program development. Japan leads the way on both counts. Having the oldest population of the seven countries which is continuing to age through the first decades of the 21st century, at the start of the new century Japan is embarking on radically new directions in policy and service delivery with the implementation of its Long-Term Care Insurance scheme in April, 2000. The articles on Japan capture the state of play in the lead up to this momentous development that is a spearhead for wider reforms in Japan's health and pension systems. The short- and longer-term outcomes will be closely monitored and evaluated not only in Japan but also in the countries of the Pacific Rim and elsewhere, as they consider options for the future of their own systems.

The articles on the United States follow. In stark contrast to Japan's highly cohesive national policies, the United States presents a picture of a "non-system" rather than a system of long-term care, defined largely with reference to the margins of the acute care system, and characterized by fragmentation and paradox. Thus, alongside the failure to resolve persistent concerns about quality of care, the success of the Programs for All-Inclusive Care of the Elderly (PACE), begun on a pilot basis in the 1970s, has provided the foundation for integrated service delivery programs across the country.

Canada provides yet another contrast. The long-term care is characterized by a relatively stable balance between national and provincial government roles that at the same time allows for considerable diversity and innovation at the local level. Upholding the national policy objectives of universal coverage and access to high quality care, is driving the search for cost effectiveness in service delivery at the provincial and local levels. Australia is also experiencing both continuity and change. Following a change of federal government in 1996, policy has continued to emphasize the expansion of community care that has applied for the previous 15 years, but recent program development has been dominated by redesign of the residential care system.

Hong Kong and Singapore at first appear similar: both are small, single-entity states, entering the 21st century on the verge of very rapid population aging, with largely Chinese value systems and family structures undergoing continuing transformations, and their economic outlooks chastened by the instability in the region at the end of the 20th century. But they also differ in approaches to financing and delivery of health care, housing, and pensions. These areas all have an important bearing on aged care, and rather than the two countries following parallel pathways as they develop their aged care systems, they will likely diverge in the future.

Finally, although Taiwan passed the marker of an aging country with 10% of its population aged 65 and over in 1995, and will not reach the level of population aging that exists in most of the other countries for at least a decade, active steps are being taken in policy and program development to prepare for that time. While Taiwan will be able to draw on the experiences of other countries, each country can learn from the others. The volume concludes with a discussion of options and lessons learned in the course of the Workshop.

In aiming to make the coverage of Pacific Rim countries in the gerontological literature available to a wide audience, the editors especially acknowledge the impact of publication of these Workshop papers in a special volume. In particular, the papers on Japan provide an update on the 1996 book on *Public Policy and the Old Age Revolution in Japan,* edited by Bass, Morris, and Oka. More generally, the focus on policy and service delivery complements the accounts of family caregiving across the East-West divide presented in the collection edited by Liu and Kendig (2000), as well as the broad-ranging surveys of demographic and social transformations associated with aging in countries at widely different levels of economic development across Asia edited by Phillips (2000).

The value of comparative study of the interconnections between long-term care policy and service delivery that this volume aims to promote could not be better expressed than in the words of Donna Yee speaking at the Workshop: "None of us knows which individuals will need long-term care, including ourselves. None of us knows if we will have the resources to get the care we might need. None of us knows how persistent and reliable we will be if we are called upon to provide long-term care for a family member or friend. Yet we each have ideas about how our society might forward needed roles and resources. This compendium of papers is an opportunity to share our notions in the context of national experiences that are culturally, economically, and politically bound to the systems under which our countries operate. Shared experiences across such boundaries can lead to creative, innovative, and effective policies and efforts to address shared challenges to care for growing populations of persons needing long-term care in each of our countries."

Iris Chi
Kalyani K. Mehta
Anna L. Howe
Editors

Long-Term Care Policy Reform in Japan

On-Kwok Lai, Dr.rer.pol

School of Policy Studies, Kwansei Gakuin University

SUMMARY. The implementation of Japan's Long-Term Care Insurance Scheme in April 2000 was the culmination of some 30 years of policy deliberation on aged care. Understanding the policy debate surrounding the Long-Term Care Insurance scheme and its financing arrangements requires an appreciation of rapid demographic and social change, especially in family structures and attitudes to caring for aged parents; but the pressures that population aging and economic downturn are placing on Japan's pension and health insurance systems also must be recognized. Even more generally, the delicate balance of political interests in Japan's central governing body, the Diet, has shaped the implementation of Long-Term Care Insurance as a forerunner to other reforms in

Dr. On-Kwok Lai is Associate Professor in Policy Studies, Kwansei Gakuin University, Japan. He received his Dr.rer.pol in Sociology/Policy from the University of Bremen, funded by the German Academic Exchange Fellowship (DAAD) in 1991. He has taught and conducted comparative research in social and public policy in Germany, Hong Kong, and New Zealand. His research interests are in comparative sociopolitical aspects of public policy, with special reference to health and welfare reform. In Spring 2000, he was visiting scholar at the Social Science Division, Hong Kong University of Science and Technology.

Dr. On-Kwok Lai can be contacted at the School of Policy Studies, Kwansei Gakuin University, Japan, 2-1 Gakuer, Sanda, Hyogo, 669-1337, Japan.

The author would like to thank the editors of this volume for their insightful comments and suggestions, and the School of Policy Studies, Kwansei Gakuin University, and the Center on Aging, The University of Hong Kong, for the financial and logistic support they provided.

[Haworth co-indexing entry note]: "Long-Term Care Policy Reform in Japan." Lai, On-Kwok. Co-published simultaneously in *Journal of Aging & Social Policy* (The Haworth Press, Inc.) Vol. 13, No. 2/3, 2001, pp. 5-20; and: *Long-Term Care in the 21st Century: Perspectives from Around the Asia-Pacific Rim* (ed: Iris Chi, Kalyani K. Mehta, and Anna L. Howe) The Haworth Press, Inc., 2001, pp. 5-20. Single or multiple copies of this article are available for a fee from The Haworth Document Delivery Service [1-800-HAWORTH, 9:00 a.m. - 5:00 p.m. (EST). E-mail address: getinfo@haworthpressinc.com].

social security and health insurance. *[Article copies available for a fee from The Haworth Document Delivery Service: 1-800-HAWORTH. E-mail address: <getinfo@haworthpressinc.com> Website: <http://www.HaworthPress.com> © 2001 by The Haworth Press, Inc. All rights reserved.]*

KEYWORDS. Family structure, financing, intergenerational transfers, long-term care insurance, policy, Japan

THE POLICY CONTEXT

The question of caring for the aging population is not a new policy discourse in Japan. For 30 years, academic, business, policy, and media reports have generated a substantial amount of knowledge, as well as policy options, for caring for the aged. Yet, because of the lack of political will–resulting from factional fights in the Liberal Democratic Party (LDP), and the political expediency for welfare populism–there has been little action. The expansionary development of health and welfare services enabled by sustained growth of the Japanese economy until recently has meant that attention has only belatedly been given to the institutional structures and policy developments needed to cope with the aging of Japanese society in general and, more specifically, for the provision of long-term care. In policy terms, it has taken more than 30 years to start the implementation of a Long-Term Care insurance (LTCI) scheme in April 2000, and it remains to be seen how long this scheme will last without some modification.

As a reminder of the uniqueness of the Japanese welfare system, we want to specify the nature of the crisis that has arisen in the system. There is no doubt that Japanese economic growth helped to create the belief that there is an alternative, Asian, model of collective welfare as compared to the European welfare state. This view was particularly the case when overseas observers witnessed the very substantial improvement of health, welfare, and quality of life achieved in Japan in the last 20 years, plus the undeniably healthy population of older Japanese. The story telling of the Japanese welfare model seemed to go unquestioned, at least until the economic crisis of the mid 1990s posed fundamental questions of financing and wastage in the health and welfare system. These questions stem from four areas in which the system has failed to respond to change: the imbalance in the share of social security funding coming from general taxation vis-à-vis premiums paid by salaried workers in the occupation-based welfare system; rapid demographic changes; changes in family structures and attitudes towards caring for the elderly; and a high-cost medical system. All these factors have had a bearing on the context in which the LTCI scheme, also known as the Nursing Care Insurance scheme, was planned from 1994 and implemented in early 2000.

The progress of the LTCI scheme has been the subject of ongoing reporting and analysis. The policy context in which proposals for the scheme emerged has been discussed in several papers in *Public Policy and the Old Age Revolution in Japan*, edited by Bass, Morris, and Oka (1996); in particular, Koyano and Shibata (1996), Okamoto (1996), and Hoshino (1996) canvass issues arising from the perspective of financing health and social care, while Adachi, Lubben, and Tsukada (1996) address the need to expand formalised in-home services. Since then, Ikegami (1997) has raised a number of problems that seemed likely to thwart implementation, but others such as Maeda (1997) and Koyano (1999) have focused on the potential of the proposed system to meet the increasingly well-recognized changes in family roles in caregiving; while the place of LTCI in the wider development of social policy for the aged has been analyzed by Usui and Palley (1997). Given this background, only a brief account of the history of the new policy is recounted here.

The Crisis of the Occupation-Based Welfare Model

After years of lagging behind some other industrial countries in providing properly coordinated social security services, the Japanese government accomplished its goal of ensuring that every member of society had a pension plan and medical insurance with the implementation of the basic framework of a national insurance scheme of social security in 1961. Once the system was established, the government was preoccupied with the task of boosting benefits in these social security programs and failed to pay due attention to future demographic changes. Aided by uninterrupted economic growth through the 1970s and 1980s, the government was able to upgrade its social security system, making such improvements as increasing pension payments, ensuring that there was no village without health and welfare services and putting in place a health insurance system for elderly people (Koseisho, 1999a/b). The Japanese welfare model seemed to work perfectly well as an accompaniment to the post-war economic miracle.

Yet, the occupation-based and labor-market financed welfare model has its limits, and as changes in the global economic climate set in, bringing regional crises and domestic problems, it reached the verge of collapse by the late 1990s. A recent statement by the Health and Welfare Ministry (Koseisho) revealed what is perhaps the true story of the Japanese welfare model, namely, that Japanese taxpayers cover a smaller portion of the bill to operate the social security system than their counterparts in the United States and Europe

(Koseisho, 1999a/b). Hence, social insurance is financed more by the contributory pensions and health insurance schemes than by various forms of general taxation, and contributions are made to all three tiers of the Japanese state-run pension system, which are:

1. The basic pension scheme sets the overall framework; it covers people in all categories of society–the self-employed, spouses of insured people, private-sector salaried workers, and government employees.
2. Corporate employees and public servants are also insured under employees' pension and mutual aid pension schemes.
3. Employees at some private-sector corporations receive benefits from funds operated by these companies.

In the late 1990s, the premiums paid by employees for their pension schemes stood at the equivalent of 17.4% of private-sector salaried workers' wages, and an average of 8.6% for health insurance. Taken together, this 25% contribution means that individual corporate workers pay the equivalent of three months' wages in premiums for their pension and health insurance plans each year, although the burden is actually split almost evenly between the employee and the employing company. Other macro data also suggest that some 65% of social security is financed by the contributory pension and health insurance schemes, and the state's monetary transfer to this sector from central and local taxes is only 25%, with the 10% balance coming from government asset investment and other income. Hence, the social insurance burden is higher than the taxation contribution.

The sustainability of the occupational welfare model is under great strain due to problems in Japan's corporate sector, including redundant workers and networking of the banking and manufacturing groups, and the need for corporate restructuring in the near future in the face of global competition and the recent Asian economic crisis. Domestically, many salaried workers already feel that they are too heavily taxed for their pension and health insurance premiums, as well as having income and other taxes deducted from their pay checks every month. The controversial consumption tax has increased from 3% when it was introduced in 1989 to 5% at present to contribute funds to welfare programs. Taxpayers may feel even harder hit if they have to pay higher premiums to meet the sharp increase in social security costs that will result from caring for an aging society in the future. The funding of social security is therefore a political as well as economic question, and the extension of the system to cover long-term care had to be done in a way that would not compound the problems of the existing system.

Rapid Demographic Change

Post-war economic growth lead to improved standards of living, including improved public hygiene and access to medical science and technology, and the average life span in Japan increased markedly. In 1947, average life expectancy was 50 years for men and 54 years for women; by 1997, these figures had risen to 77 for men and 84 for women, increases of 27 years and 30 years, respectively, in the 50-year period. Average life expectancy in Japan is now the highest in the world.

The size of the elderly population is increasing sharply as life span increases. The 65 and older population increased from 4.16 million in 1950 to 21.87 million in 2000, more than a four-fold increase over this 50-year period. The increase in the population of the old-old (75 and older) was particularly marked, increasing from 1.07 million to 7 million, a 6.5-fold increase, in the same period (NIPS, 2000).

Several features of Japan's demographic aging warrant particular note. First, aging is a comparatively recent phenomenon in Japan, beginning only in the 1970s. Second, Japan is the most rapidly aging society in the world; by 2000, it had the highest proportion of population aged 65 and over of any country, 17%, and this figure will reach 22% by 2010, with Japan maintaining its global lead for another 50 years. Third, the number of the old-old will continue to increase ahead of the total aged population; compared to just a third of the total aged population in 2000, the old-old will account for close to half of the elderly in 2010, 10.5 million out of 28.13 million. Fourth, by 2020, some one-in-three families across the country will be headed by elderly people, and from 2000 to 2020, over half of the elderly will be in single-person or couple-only households (NIPS, 2000). Finally, based on the medium projections in the Population Projections for Japan of the National Institute of Population and Social Security Research (NIPS, 1997), the proportion of aged will reach 26% in 2020 (about 32.3 million), and will continue to rise to an initial peak of 28% in 2030, and peak again at 32% around 2050 (NIPS, 2000). With one out of every four citizens aged 65 and over, and one in two of these aged 75 and over, the 21st century in Japan is truly the "century of the elderly."

Changing Family Structures and Attitudes
Towards Supporting the Elderly

The transformation of the family in post-war Japan has had the greatest impact on the elderly. As society has grown increasingly oriented toward nuclear families, the percentage of households where children and the elderly live under the same roof has been decreasing. In 1960, over 85% of the elderly lived with their children, but this figure is now just over half; conversely, single-person elderly households that accounted for only 5.4% in 1960 have increased to 17% in 2000, and another 28% were then couples-only households compared to 7% in 1960.

These changes reflect increasing standards of living of both older and younger people, and rural to urban shifts of younger people, and are made all the more significant by the high rate of marriage and, hence, lower rate of single-person households due to non-marriage, compared to western countries. The decline in co-residence has occurred despite a number of aspects of the Taxation Exemption Allowances and Employment Benefit (Special Allowance), which can influence decisions about taking parent(s) or parents-in-law into the Family Account on which taxation is based. Co-residence is also reinforced by the Household Registration System at the local government level and the multi-generation mortgage arrangement available in the property market for home purchase.

With the demographic trends of fewer children and an aging population, coupled with the economic problems that Japan is experiencing, attitudes toward supporting elderly parents and aged relatives are also changing markedly. A nation-wide survey by the Ministry of Health and Welfare in 1994 found that 60% of the caregivers thought their burden was too great. It is becoming increasingly difficult to expect that families will provide full support for their elderly, and the problems of illness and long-term care have been identified as the greatest concern of the elderly (Campbell & Ikegami, 1999; Koseisho, 1999a/b).

The economic uncertainties that the younger generations must face, including less secure job tenure, having to be ready for more mobile job locations, and the dual roles of women in the family and the workforce, mean they are beginning to think about living together with their parents and supporting their parents in need of care as separate issues. In the past, living together with parents has implied caring for them, but now many younger people, especially daughters and daughters-in-law, are looking to ways of providing care for their parents that do not involve co-residence.

In addition to the dynamics of population aging outlined above, a number of other economic and social issues must be addressed. First, even though some 60% of the elderly are economically dependent on the pension system, there is a large income differential among elderly households, so that low-income elderly require more financial support from their families. Second, there is a tension between the trend to early retirement versus the wish to work post-retirement. Third, caring for the elderly is increasingly seen as a shared responsibility of public services and private families, and a responsibility that should be shared more equitably between men and women. Fourth, by 2020, over half the elderly will be living alone or with an elderly spouse only.

High-Cost Medical Care

The aging question was well articulated by the Council on Population in a report in August 1969 that highlighted that the world's lowest birth rate would make Japan an "elderly nation" in 30 years. Those 30 years have passed since the Council's advisory panel made its recommendations to the Health and Welfare Ministry, but not much has been done by way of actual policy change and systematic reform. Those years also saw the political expediency of holding on to voters' loyalty combined with the powerful professional interests such as the Japan Medical Association, which literally blocked any reform initiative for health cost containment. Together these influences reinforced the further development and expansion of health and welfare programs with little recognition that the system was defaulting on aging.

One of the synergistic effects of the pro-growth approach in health and welfare has been the development of a very high-technology, high-cost medical system. Clinics and hospitals, whether privately or publicly funded, tend to be costly and high-technology based. Overseas visitors are surprised to see the latest medical equipment being placed in ordinary clinics. On the other hand, users of inpatient services appear to stay longer than in other countries, but this is in part because of the unclear separation of acute hospitals from long-stay and rehabilitation hospitals.

Although health care accounts for a low share of Japan's GDP (Gross Domestic Product) compared to other OECD countries, the rate of increase has been higher; the 7.5% share in 2000 was up from 6% in 1990, and per capita outlays increased by almost 40% over the decade. Further, internal transfers are now critical to staving off bankruptcy of the health insurance schemes, and funds for the health sector from both government and individual households are shrinking. The first attempt at cost-containment in four decades, the Health Insurance Law implemented in 1997 to lower the rate of increase for the overall health care expenditure, was not successful, and the high-cost health care sector is still inefficiently run. The compounding effect of aging on the cost of medical and hospital care is already evident.

Approaching 40% of the total expenditure of ¥30 trillion[1] will probably go to covering medical and hospital expenses for patients aged 65 and over in fiscal 1999-2000 (*Mainichi Daily News,* February 8, 2000). In age cohorts terms, medical bills incurred by aged people are five times greater than those still contributing and working regularly. The impending growth in medical and hospital expenditures is one of the prime reasons for separating out the costs of long-term care and transferring them to the LTCI scheme. As this scheme draws on other sources of funding, it can assist in containing the premiums to be paid for health insurance.

POLICY OBJECTIVES OF STRUCTURAL REFORM

The social security system in Japan covers five major areas: medical and health care, social welfare, pensions, employment and related insurance, and public hygiene. Its main policy objective is to protect the whole population's health and welfare, but it has not until now made special provision for long-term care. Facing an aging population with fewer children, and a proportionately smaller workforce, the 1990s was a period for structural reform of social security programs. That the LTCI scheme has been the first initiative to be implemented indicates both the priority of long-term care, and that it has been easier, or at least less difficult, to introduce a new scheme than to modify the existing schemes in other areas.

The Japanese Model of Financing Social Security

Following interest repayments for national debt, social security is the largest single item in the government's budget; expenditure of ¥16,095 billion accounted for 19.7% of the total budget in 1999. Fully 65% of social security inputs in Japan are financed by contributory premiums for pensions and health insurance. A main policy goal is to reduce this share to 50% and have the other 50% provided by other forms of taxation.

The Japanese taxation system has three major financial implications for funding social expenditures. First, the tax base and the volume of direct tax derived from salaried workers is relatively small; indirect taxes and the consumption tax thus have an important role to play for funding new programs. Second, for the majority of salaried households, the tax contribution is less than the social insurance contributions paid for pensions and health insurance, at a ratio of 1:1.3. Third, the balance between social insurance and taxation is inversely proportional to income; for lower-income households, the social insurance burden is high in proportion to the tax burden, while higher-income households contribute more through taxes compared to social insurance contributions.

Turning to outlays, and taking fiscal year 1996 as an example, the balance of social security expenditure was 52% on pensions and 37% on medical services, with the balance on other areas (Koseisho, 1999a; Ito, 1999). More importantly, payments to the elderly population accounted for 64% of the total budget, with a 3:1 ratio for outlays on pensions to health care. As the aging momentum increases, there will be increasing pressure on these payments. Even in the short term, the consumption tax will have to rise to 7% from the present 5% if the existing level of outlays on programs for the elderly is to be maintained until the year 2005. The introduction of the consumption tax in 1989 coincided with moves to expand long-term care services, especially community care, and facilitated this growth, but only postponed rather than obviated the need for further reform for financing long-term care.

The Golden Plan and the New Golden Plan

Concerted action to expand the range of services available for long-term care of the elderly was first taken in 1989, with the introduction of the Ten-Year Strategy to Promote Health Care and Welfare for the Elderly, known as the Golden Plan. The Golden Plan was established to achieve integrated development of health, medical care, and welfare for the elderly over a 10-year period, and aimed to implement a service system that would allow elderly people requiring long-term care to be as independent as possible and continue to live in their accustomed homes and communities. Under the Plan, in-home services especially were expanded, but institutional welfare services were also enhanced and rehabilitation services were expanded to prevent elderly patients from becoming bedridden. In 1990, administration of welfare services was shifted to the municipalities, and the establishment of a Local Health and Welfare Plan for the Elderly in each municipality became mandatory. Funding for these long-term care services continued to be through the welfare and health components of the social security system, bolstered by the new consumption tax.

In 1994, to meet expanded needs arising from the implementation of the Golden Plan, the New Golden Plan was introduced and laid the foundation on which long-term care services for the elderly were to be built. Again, there were no reforms to financing.

Financing Reform

Establishment of a social insurance scheme for financing long-term care was first put forward for discussion in December 1994 in a "Report on Nursing Care for the Elderly and a Supportive System for Independence" and was further recommended by the Social Security System Review Council in July 1995. After gaining support from three major political parties, the Bill was tabled for Diet discussion in November 1996. The Nursing Care Insurance Law was enacted on December 17, 1997 (Hiramatsu, 1999; Koseisho, 1999a/b; Mi-

nerva Shobou, 1999). The LTCI Law has 14 chapters and 215 rules, and is sup-
plemented by the LTCI Implementation Law, which has another 19 rules. The
structure of this legislation is similar to the 12 major laws that govern the provision of other welfare services under the Japanese Constitution (Matsui,
1999) and the administration of services at the municipal level. These laws and
their subsidiary by-laws are very detailed and specify service standards and
protocols, staffing, and administrative responsibilities of provider agencies.
The laws covering the LTCI scheme are thus highly consistent with the existing legislative infrastructure, although the long-term care scheme itself has introduced major changes in service delivery and financing.

As a first step towards structural reform of the social security system to
cope with rapid population aging, the new insurance scheme is bringing about
a large-scale reorganization of the long-term care system, which until now has
been divided into welfare services and medical care services. The new scheme
also aims to create an efficient and fair social support system. To this end, the
dual key considerations are to build steadily on the foundation of long-term
care services and create an insurance-based financing system for long-term
care. The goals of the LTCI scheme are as follows:

- To provide a care system in which users can freely choose services;
- To offer welfare and medical care services related to long-term care in a
  unified and integrated manner;
- To provide diversified and efficient services through the participation of
  entities such as private businesses and non-profit organizations; and
- To rectify the long stays in general hospitals for reasons of long-term
  care (so-called "social hospitalization") and create more efficient medical services.

In undertaking these reforms as part of the wider reform of the social security system, there must be consensus among the general public. The overriding
considerations that must be kept in mind in this regard are achieving higher efficiency overall through reorganization across programs, ensuring user-ori-
ented services with higher efficiency, and ensuring fairness, equity, and
equality across the social divides of generations, gender, and income.

These considerations underlie the reforms that have been proposed for each
part of the system, separately and collectively, across the system (Koseisho,
1999a/b). The LTCI scheme has led the way in implementation; the other reforms are in the process of implementation or under consideration. Gradual reform of medical insurance has been implemented from 1997 to increase
efficiency of medical care while ensuring its quality. Beginning with attempts
to control rising insurance premiums and introduce pricing mechanisms, the

reforms have moved into the entire range of the medical care delivery and medical insurance system, while maintaining universal coverage. Comprehensive reform is, however, yet to come, particularly on the basic issues of who finances medical care and the levels of benefits.

In the area of public pensions, the system overall is being reviewed to achieve appropriate levels of benefits without causing the burden to become excessive in the future, while taking into account the balance between the level of benefits and that of real income for the future generations. Proposals with draft legislation are being studied by the Diet, and the related legislative changes will take place from 2000 to 2005.

For welfare services other than long-term care for the elderly, a new service delivery system must be developed. A Plan for People with Disabilities was drawn up in 1995, aimed at achieving rehabilitation and normalization in the community. Action is needed to promote integration across programs and establish comprehensive measures that will provide a livelihood support system for people with disabilities.

Financing Arrangements for the LTCI Scheme

The LTCI scheme is a social insurance scheme in so far as premiums are collected and risks shared across the whole population, but it is not a funded insurance scheme; that is, current premiums pay for current costs rather than providing for the cost of future use of long-term care on the part of those who now pay premiums. The financing arrangements involve cost sharing and co-payments so that no single source of funding is over-burdened.

Cost sharing. The overall budget of the LTCI scheme was estimated at ¥4.2 trillion at the start of the scheme in April 2000, when there were expected to be over 2.8 million certified users. It is jointly funded by policy owners' premium payments and government funds, each making up 50% of the fund.

Of the 50% premium income from the insured population, 17% will come from those in Category 1 (aged 65 or above) and 33% from those in Category 2 (aged 40 to 64). The remaining 50% will be contributed by all three levels of government: prefectural governments and local municipalities will each contribute 12.5%, and the central government will provide 25%, of which 5% is an adjustable contribution to compensate for regional differentials in age-weighting for local municipalities. In addition, there will be a stability fund set up within the tripartite government framework to cope with possible increases in long-term care expenditure or to cover unpaid or non-recoverable premium contributions. Each government party is responsible for one-third of this fund.

Premiums. The method of premium payments for 70%-80% of the elderly in Category 1 is expected as deductions from the pension payments they receive, automatically charged through the pension system. The remaining 20%-30% will pay directly to the municipal LTCI office. For the younger age groups in Category 2, the premium payment will be added to their health insurance and then channelled to the municipality (Asahi, 1999; Koseisho, 1999a/b). Payment of the premiums is integrated with existing social security infrastructure and achieves efficiencies in not requiring a separate financial infrastructure.

The monthly premium of those 65 and above is estimated at a national average of ¥2,915 at the start of the scheme. The premium payments are set on a five-step scale following the taxation status of the insured. The standard premium is ¥3,000 per month at step 3, for those with no taxable income per month, with adjustments of 25% up and down. Thus, those who have least income (protected household/welfare pension recipients) will have to pay only 50% of the standard premium, while there will be two higher steps for those paying tax, to a maximum of 150% of step 3. It is expected that unless there is major re-categorization, the premium level will stay the same for three years.

Co-payments. Generally speaking, service recipients are charged 10% of the cost of services, plus food costs.

Effect on Cost Containment and Cost Recovery

The implementation of the LTCI scheme will undoubtedly bring a significant improvement for central, prefectural, and local governments in the fiscal management of long-term care for the elderly and others in need of long-term care.

At the macro level, the systematic design of the LTCI scheme is obviously aiming for cost containment and shifting costs for long-term care from the medical and health care budget to the newly established LTCI budget. It also aims to foster quasi-competitive market conditions by admitting more and different suppliers of services, with a view to achieving cost efficiency and innovation. More importantly, in light of the sharp growth in social security costs in the foreseeable future, the government has asked elderly people to shoulder a share of the burden in proportion to their income through the LTCI premiums.

The LTCI scheme, however, has not fully addressed the medical needs of the aged, nor the cost implications of medical expenses of acute care for the aged. Among the controversial issues that have yet to be explored are whether the aged will continue to be entitled to the same acute care coverage as other age groups, or whether the LTCI is to be complemented by an effort to have elderly people pay a fixed rate of fees for acute treatment and medicines they receive, with an upper limit set on the bill to be shouldered by such patients.

At the meso level, there are built-in mechanisms to contain the cost of long-term care. At the local and regional levels, the insured, on the one hand, will have to deal with service providers directly under the terms and conditions laid down by the local authority. On the other hand, standardized costing for contracted types of services under the LTCI scheme should give local and prefectural government considerable leverage to adjust the level, quantity, and quality of the service supplied.

At the micro level, the means to cost containment lie in the practice of classification of levels of care, using both computerized and professional screening and assessment, and regular review. The gate-keeping or rationing role of the care managers will at the same time guarantee and limit the supply of the scheduled services. Any services over and above the standardized or recommended levels will have to be paid for by the service users.

THE INCOMPLETE LONG-TERM CARE PROJECT: PENSION REFORM AHEAD

Good policy and financing for long-term care are not just about enhancing life expectancy for the elderly; they are also about ensuring the quality of life they can enjoy. To this end, it is fundamentally important that medical and health care should be anchored in economic and social security; it is here that the question of stability of the social security system needs to be addressed.

Prospects for Pension Reform

The present arrangements for financing social security for Japan's aging society have an inter-generational gap with reference to contributions and benefits. To many elderly people, the pension system is a basic financial resource for their remaining days. However, both middle-aged and younger people have become disaffected with the state-run pension system. Middle-aged people are concerned that they may receive less than they have paid, while younger people are reluctant to shoulder a heavy burden in the form of premiums now and in the future.

The greatest challenge facing Japan is to address the normative and ethical issues of policy on aging: the fundamental questions are who should pay, and how much, to finance the pension, medical, and LTCI systems. Since there is every reason to believe that the total cost of these systems will become greater year by year, the more the political delay and indecision, the worse the financial conditions will be. Reform, therefore, should not focus only on social security, but also on the taxation regime. One proposal mooted by the main opposition party (Democratic Party) was to increase the consumption tax to 7% or to use it exclusively for welfare programs for the elderly. While this proposal solves the inter-generational problems of financing, it generates questions of the redistributive justice of indirect taxation.

In late 1999, a government-sponsored bill was submitted to the Diet to reform the pension system. The bill would increase the ratio of premiums to be covered by state subsidies from one-third to one-half, after ensuring that the government finds stable means of raising funds. While this bill would address the risk of the collapse of the pension system, no new policy could be implemented until the end of 2004 at the earliest, assuming there were no more political blockages in the legislative process. So the prospect for pension reform remains uncertain.

Inertia and Administrative-Political Deadlock

In 1997, the Health and Welfare Ministry unveiled five options for reforming the state-run pension system. According to the Ministry, the government would have to raise the premiums paid by corporate employees for their pension plans to a hefty 34.3% of their monthly salaries by 2025 if they were to receive benefits comparable with the current levels. The five options represented an attempt by the ministry to provide the public with food for thought concerning whether they should choose an increase in the premiums they would have to pay, or cuts in benefits they would receive.

But there is inertia and administrative-political deadlock for the overhaul of the crisis-ridden social security system. In the late 1990s, Japanese bureaucrats, their intelligent images tarnished by various scandals, had yet to overcome the problem of the lack of coordination among ministries and over-coordination of intra-ministerial programs. The resultant clannish mindset limits the capacity of all institutions concerned to work toward mutually shared goals.

In the political arena, few politicians dare take steps to implement cuts in pensions and other social security benefits, or increase the financial burden to be shouldered by the public, for fear of losing votes. Welfare populism remains the currency for securing political position, particularly in a climate of more multi-party politics. In addition, none of the organizations with a stake in social security programs, such as the Japan Medical Association, health insurance associations, business organizations and labor unions, stands ready to abandon its vested interests. This has led to a gridlock among the parties concerned, just when the need to take action for reform is most urgent.

Political Compromise and Lack of Political Will

A final twist in the political road to implementation of the LTCI scheme, if not a U-turn, was that an election had to be held before October 2000. In the lead up to the election that was held on June 26, the ruling coalition in the Diet election adopted the tactic of delaying the introduction of the LTCI premium contribution to be paid by the elderly population. The tactic worked, and despite losing 60 seats, the Liberal Democratic Party (LDP) returned as the leader of the ruling coalition of the Liberal Party and New Komeito, and maintains the majority in the Diet.

But the new political packaging of the revised LTCI scheme with the so-called six-month "grace period" for the premium from the aged and cash options for family carers, coupled with a review six months after the LTCI scheme was implemented, angered the public and many municipal officials. Their fear was that the very spirit of the LTCI scheme would be compromised, if not jeopardized, for partisan politics. Even more problematic is building political consensus for further reforms, which will be more difficult to achieve as a result of the Diet election, which further strengthened the opposition forces inside and outside the Diet.

The politically fragile ruling parties sidestepped the aging question and the funding of long-term care needs by their decision to delay collecting premiums in the hopes of wooing voters. They appear oblivious to the need to improve the foundations of the scheme and to come up with stable sources of operating funds–both tasks that should be undertaken from a long-term perspective. Welfare populism again triumphed over political will to develop policies addressing the basic principles of inter-generational, horizontal, and vertical transfers of tax and insurance burdens. In political economy terms, the struggle for sustainable and healthy long-term care is just beginning.

NOTE

1. Note on currency. Throughout this paper, yen is used because of the fluctuating exchange rate of the yen against the US dollar; the rate was ¥149 in August 1998, ¥102 in December 1999, and about ¥108 in July 2000.

REFERENCES

Adachi, K., Lubben, J. E., & Tsukada, N. (1996). Expansion of formalized in-home services for Japan's aged. In Bass, S. A., Morris, R., & Oka, M. (Eds.) (1996). *Public Policy and the Old Age Revolution in Japan*. New York: The Haworth Press, Inc. 147-160.
Asahi, Kenji. (1999). *Kaigohoken no Point* [Points of Long Tern Care Insurance]. Tokyo: Kiri Shobo.
Campbell, J. C., & Ikegami, N. (1999). *Long Term Care for Frail Older People: Reaching for the Ideal Solution*. Keio University Symposium for Life Science and Medicine, vol. 4. Tokyo: Springer-Verlag.

Hiramatsu, K. (1999). *Kagohoken Service* [Long Term Care Service]. Tokyo: Dental-Medico-Pharmaceutical Publishers.

Hoshino, S. (1996). Paying for the health and social care of the elderly. In Bass, S. A., Morris, R., & Oka, M. (Eds.) (1996). *Public Policy and the Old Age Revolution in Japan.* New York: The Haworth Press, Inc. 37-56.

Ikegami, N. (1997). Public long-term care insurance in Japan. *Journal of the American Medical Association, 278*: 1310-1314.

Ito, Shuhei. (1997). *Kaigohoken.* [Long Term Care Insurance]. Tokyo: Aoki-Shoten.

Koseisho [Ministry of Health & Welfare]. (1999a). *Kosei* [Health & Welfare] White Paper. Tokyo: Koseisho.

Koseisho [Ministry of Health & Welfare]. (1999b). *Shakkai Fukushi no Direction* [Direction of Social Welfare]. Tokyo: Koseisho.

Koyano, W. (1999). Population aging, changes in living arrangement, and the new long-term care system in Japan. *Journal of Sociology and Social Welfare, 26*: 155-167.

Koyano, W., & Shibata, H. (1996). The health status of elderly people and the new direction of health services. In Bass, S. A., Morris, R., & Oka, M. (Eds.) (1996), *Public Policy and the Old Age Revolution in Japan.* New York: The Haworth Press, Inc. 13-24.

Maeda, D. (1997). Work and eldercare in Japan. *Japanese Journal of Social Science, 1*(5): 64.

Mainichi Daily News (2000). February 8.

Matsui, S. (1999). *Nihonkoku kempou* [Japan Constitution]. Tokyo: Yuhi-kaku.

Minerva, S. (1999). *Shakkai Fukuishi Shoropou* [Six Laws on Social Welfare]. Tokyo: Minerva Shobou.

National Institute of Population and Social Security Research [NIPS] (1997). *Population Projections for Japan: 1996-2050 and 2051-2100.* Research Series No. 291, April 1997. Tokyo: NIPS.

National Institute of Population and Social Security Research [NIPS] (2000). *Household Projections for Japan by Prefecture: 1995-2050.* Research Series No. 298, March 2000. Tokyo: NIPS.

Okamoto, A. (1996). Japan's financing system for health care of the elderly. In Bass, S. A., Morris, R., & Oka, M. (Eds.) (1996), *Public Policy and the Old Age Revolution in Japan.* New York: The Haworth Press, Inc. 25-36.

Takao, Yusuo. (1999). Welfare state retrenchment–The case of Japan. *Journal of Public Policy, 19*(3): 265-292.

Usui, C., & Palley, H. A. (1997). The development of social policy for the elderly in Japan. *Social Services Review, 71*: 360-381.

Aged Care Service Delivery in Japan: Preparing for the Long-Term Care Insurance Scheme

Ritsuko Watanabe, PhD
On-Kwok Lai, Dr.rer.pol

School of Policy Studies, Kwansei Gakuin University

SUMMARY. The implementation of Japan's Long-Term Care Insurance Scheme in early 2000 presaged many changes in service delivery and much debate among service providers, different levels of government, academic analysts, and major media interests. The first part of this paper gives an account of the major changes in the organization of service

Dr. Ritsuko Watanabe is Professor at the School of Policy Studies, Kwansei Gakuin University. Dr. Watanabe received her PhD in Social Welfare from the University of Michigan in 1990. She is the recipient of the France Bed Foundation Research Award and New York State New Faculty Development Award.

Dr. On-Kwok Lai is Associate Professor in Policy Studies, Kwansei Gakuin University, Japan. He received his Dr.rer.pol in Sociology/Policy from the University of Bremen, funded by the German Academic Exchange Fellowship (DAAD) in 1991. He has taught and conducted comparative research in social and public policy in Germany, Hong Kong, and New Zealand. His research interests are in comparative sociopolitical aspects of public policy, with special reference to health and welfare reform. In Spring 2000, he was visiting scholar at the Social Science Division, Hong Kong University of Science and Technology.

Both authors can be contacted at the School of Policy Studies, Kwansei Gakuin University, Japan, 2-1 Gakuer, Sanda, Hyogo, 669-1337, Japan (Dr. On-Kwok Lai's E-mail: oklai@ksc.kwansei.ac.jp; Dr. Ritsuko Watanabe's E-mail: z95039@ksc.kwansei.ac.jp).

[Haworth co-indexing entry note]: "Aged Care Service Delivery in Japan: Preparing for the Long-Term Care Insurance Scheme." Watanabe, Ritsuko, and On-Kwok Lai. Co-published simultaneously in *Journal of Aging & Social Policy* (The Haworth Press, Inc.) Vol. 13, No. 2/3, 2001, pp. 21-34; and: *Long-Term Care in the 21st Century: Perspectives from Around the Asia-Pacific Rim* (ed: Iris Chi, Kalyani K. Mehta, and Anna L. Howe) The Haworth Press, Inc., 2001, pp. 21-34. Single or multiple copies of this article are available for a fee from The Haworth Document Delivery Service [1-800-HAWORTH, 9:00 a.m. - 5:00 p.m. (EST). E-mail address: getinfo@haworthpressinc.com].

delivery that have increased opportunities for private sector providers, including large corporations, and restructured contractual relationships between municipalities and providers in all sectors. New arrangements for client assessment, classification, care management, and extended service types are then outlined. An assessment is then made of the likelihood that the expected outcomes of the scheme will be realized, with the concerns of welfare professionals that the public welfare system is under threat juxtaposed with bureaucratic goals of liberalizing the provision of long-term care. *[Article copies available for a fee from The Haworth Document Delivery Service: 1-800-HAWORTH. E-mail address: <getinfo@haworthpressinc.com> Website: <http://www.HaworthPress.com> © 2001 by The Haworth Press, Inc. All rights reserved.]*

KEYWORDS. Assessment, classification, care management, Japan, Long-Term Care Insurance

ORGANIZATION OF LONG-TERM CARE

This paper covers the development of the long-term care service delivery system in Japan up to the implementation of the Long-Term Care Insurance scheme on April 1, 2000. The new system commenced on that date, apart from the collection of premiums to be paid by the insured population, which was delayed for six months. Long-Term Care Insurance is the first of a set of comprehensive policy reforms tackling different issues of population aging in Japan and focuses on those who need assistance in daily living and particularly those who are bedridden.

The new scheme covers a wide range of both community care and institutional care services. The scheme is commonly known as "nursing care insurance" as well as Long-Term Care Insurance in Japan, reflecting the need for nursing care as the base requirement for eligibility for all services covered by the scheme. In this paper, we use the term "Long-Term Care Insurance" (LTCI) for the scheme, "long-term care" when referring to the wider range of services, and "nursing care" for care services provided by nurses.

Service Administration and Selection of Service Providers

The LTCI scheme is attempting to build up a 24-hour, all-round service delivery system at the community level, administered by the local municipalities, with local service providers in the quasi-public and private sectors, that is, non-profit and profit-making bodies (Asahi, 1999; Komuro & Nagatani, 1999). To promote efficiency of the system overall, built-in mechanisms promote care alternatives to residential care, as well as competition for quality improvement, within a given standardized set of certified services.

While administration of the LTCI scheme builds on existing infrastructure by way of municipal-based service planning and delivery, changes to the arrangement have been required, and a number of new features have been introduced. In contrast to the tripartite funding arrangements that involve central, prefectural, and local governments, health and welfare services in Japan are mostly administered and delivered by the local municipalities. The functions of the prefectural level of government in Japan are broadly equivalent to state or provincial governments in other federal systems. The role of municipalities was strengthened from 1994, and they deliver services usually with joint financial and policy coordination with the prefectural government and central government ministerial agencies (Takao, 1999).

Although the LTCI system has been centrally developed at the ministry level and is "top-down" in managerial terms, actual service delivery is more decentralized, and the locally autonomous governance structure allows for local municipalities to develop alternative plans and legal protocols within an overall national framework (Matsui, 1999; Minerva, 1999). The national framework sets some conditions, such as the range of services to be covered by LTCI and the premiums to be paid by those aged 40 to 64 years, but local government has to decide the premiums for the elderly and also whether to provide extra services, such as meals, which are not included in the LTCI scheme. Thus, there will be some variations around a central model in each of the 47 Prefectures, 17 Special Designated Cities (like Kobe and Osaka), and 3,252 municipalities (cities, districts, and villages) since they must develop their own protocols for the LTCI scheme.

The most radical departures from the old system are the entry of new service providers in the burgeoning nursing care market and the new contractual relationship between these providers and consumers.

Growth and Differentiation of Service Providers

The total number of registered nursing care providers increased by 55% when the new scheme was implemented, with 196,221 providers registered at the end of April 2000 compared to 126,071 in March 2000 (*Kaigohoken Monthly*, June 2000, p. 22). Most of the increase is derived from private providers seeking to enter the nursing care market as new suppliers, with three main kinds of new providers emerging. First, large-scale corporations that already had nursing services and were sending home-helpers or visiting nurses to families, were enlarging this type of service, knowing LTCI would shortly be in place. Second, large-scale corporations that have never provided long-term care services have developed this business and have recently opened many branches in local areas, as well as smaller operating units in remote areas. Third, not-for-profit organizations or small-scale business enterprises that have provided inexpensive home help services have registered.

There are now four distinct providers groups. In rank order of their respective contributions in the field, the largest are medical, nursing, and allied health professionals based in clinics and hospitals, which account for up to 60% of nursing and allied health care for the aged. This group constitutes most of the nursing services in terms of number of organizations, and some have special taxation status. The next largest group are municipal-sponsored and funded service providers, which grew considerably in the expansionary welfare-populism era but which are expected to have a decreasing role as their share of provision is seen to be under threat, and their survival in light of the recent reforms is a topic of considerable debate. Welfare foundations that are legally incorporated bodies are an historic form of welfare agency and will play a small role since some will shift to non-profit status if they can attract support under the LTCI scheme. Non-profit organizations that operate under the new law enacted in 1998 governing non-profit organizations can also be included in this group; their roles have expanded. The most recent entrants in the field have come from a strong national movement of volunteerism, partly resulting from the Hansin-Awaji earthquake in 1995. Finally, private, profit-making businesses providing welfare services are seen as having the potential to gain a larger market share because of their large corporation financing and aggressive marketing. It remains to be seen whether their role does in fact eventuate on a large scale as some of these private businesses have already withdrawn from home-helper or care-management services because they were not sufficiently profitable and because clients tended to choose municipal-sponsored services more because they had a long history of service delivery before the LTCI scheme.

New contractual relationships between service providers and users. The most important structural change is the new set of contractual relationships between (a) the municipality and the insured, (b) the insured and the care service providers, and (c) the care service providers with the municipality. In the previous arrangements for care service for the aged, the municipalities commissioned the service providers and the latter provided service for the aged. The municipalities mostly assumed the commissioned providers could do the whole job efficiently, from screening and assessment to providing all kinds of services. However, there was the possibility of under- or over- provision in relation to the target needs, and cost was less likely contained because the commitment for the aged was open-ended (Komuro & Nagatani, 1999).

Under the new scheme, the basic relationship between the municipality and the client is an insurance one, that is, a public contractual relationship governed by the LTCI Law. The insured have a limited entitlement and the insuring agency, namely government, offers a premium-conditioned supply of entitlements; municipal governments also have the assessment/screening function of understanding and planning for the needs of their aged populations but can shape the demand side of the long-term care market by capping the entitlement.

Potentially more significant developments are the new, private, contractual relationships between the different service providers and the insured clients, who are free to choose their service providers, type, and quality of services. This relationship is intended to create a market-oriented system through enhancing customers' choices on the demand side and promoting efficiency of providers on the supply side. In addition, the insuring agency of the municipalities can also influence the standardized costing/pricing of the suppliers; present costing favors the profit-making long-term care providers because the profit margin between the pricing and cost (labor in particular) is quite large. This margin was intended to attract more private providers and so expand provision, but customers are learning that they cannot afford to use highly priced services to satisfy their service needs within the limit of LTCI. One way in which customers are making cost-effective use of the LTCI funding is by purchasing only the cheaper services, such as homemaking, instead of personal care services.

Further, non-profit providers have benefited from this pricing and have expanded their operations, making it harder for new private providers to enter the field. Since non-profit providers tend to provide cheaper service to compete with the private providers, more customers are choosing these cheaper services within the given LTCI coverage. The provision of high-priced care services by the private profit-making providers has not met a good response from the limited LTCI funded customers, and the private sector is not expanding as much as expected, with many of the potential for-profit suppliers now taking a "wait and see" position. The outcome of the pricing and the limited amount of LTCI coverage has tended to be an increase in the supply of low-cost, low-quality long-term care services.

Classification of Clients for LTCI Entitlements and Pricing

After screening and certification for nursing care needs, service users will be placed in one of the six care levels. These levels are described as 1 + 5, with a base level of general support and five graduated levels of increasing funding related to care needs. The Care Ranks, funding levels, and typical service mixes at each level are detailed in Table 1.

The quantity and types of recommended services differ according to the category of need, with the service charge (unit costing) usually reflecting the level of service complexity and the time factor. More specifically, the pricing of the 1 + 5 levels of LTCI entitlement to care services is based on the standardized time-input for providing nursing care. The lowest level is ¥64,000 per month, and the highest is about ¥368,000 per month. In actual operation, the entitlement in terms of the LTCI Care Rank can be seen as a sort of coupon that gives the certified client a means of expressing his or her demand in the nursing care market. Clients can choose a package of services within the purchasing power of the entitlement, or if they want more services above the entitlement level, they can pay for the excess.

In November 1999, the three parties in the central government agreed to a cash alternative to service provision. This cash alternative will make it possible to pay up to ¥100,000 a month, plus an unspecified amount of non-cash contribution, to families caring for elders certified as eligible for long-term care services on condition that they do not receive a nursing service. In some circumstances, it may also be possible for families to cash in the entitlement to care services to take care of their relative who is certified LTCI-eligible. While these cash options could offer an alternative in municipalities where services have not developed sufficiently to meet all needs, the decision to allow the options was not well received by many municipal officers since it could undermine local service development. It is not known how far elderly people and their families will prefer cash to services.

Care Managers and the Care Plan

Before recipients receive nursing care from the mostly private providers, they will have a professional consultation with an accredited and qualified Care Manager, resulting in a Care Plan detailing the course of action, timing, and cost, etc. (Komuro & Nagatani, 1999; KK, 1999; Yamamoto, 1999). Many professionals and paraprofessionals who have several years of practice can obtain Care Manager's Qualification, via a state examination. Along with doctors, nurses, physiotherapists, occupational therapists, and social workers, other groups, such as acupuncturists, have qualified, and the diversity of backgrounds and training of the qualified Care Managers is now causing many problems. Problems are especially evident in differences in Care Managers' assessments and decisions on services to be provided to LTCI recipients.

TABLE 1. Example of the Certified Care-Rank and Care-Rating System

Care-Rank Level	Maximum Service Fee Paid by Government (10% paid by service user)	Example of Typical Service Combination and Service Frequencies (No. per Week)
General Support	¥64,000 (less than US$640)	2 Day service visits
Care Level 1	¥170,000	1 Home help service visit 1 Visiting nurse visit 3 Day service visits
Care Level 2	¥201,000	3 Home help service visits 1 Visiting nurse visit 3 Day service visits
Care Level 3	¥274,000	2 Home help service visits 1 Visiting nurse visit 7 Rotating visiting nurse visits 3 Day service visits
Care Level 4	¥323,000	6 Home help service visits 2 Visiting nurse visits 7 Rotating visiting nurse visits 1 Day service visit
Care Level 5	¥368,000	6 Home help service visits 2 Visiting nurse visits 1 VRPV 14 Rotating visiting nurse visits

The Care Plan will normally be reviewed at six-month intervals. The type of care that a recipient will receive is determined by the local government-accredited Care Managers, and more often than not, Care Managers also assume the role of screening and assessing the elderly for the certification of their Care Rank. The role of Care Manager and the Care Plan are thus both of critical importance; they are instrumental in providing a better information base to help the insured choose among various competing care providers and to shop around with the given entitlements on the one hand and enhancing the quality of nursing services on the other.

SERVICE DELIVERY

Target Users

The size of the aged population who need the services to be provided under the LTCI scheme was estimated at 2.8 million in 2000. This estimate means that 16% of the entire senior population are expected to become users of some kind of long-term care service at the start of the system.

The LTCI scheme covers all those aged 40 and above, but this total target population is divided in two groups: Category 1–aged 65 and above, and Category 2–aged 40 to 64. Individuals in both groups will be prescribed long-term care services if they have been certified after screening and assessment.

Assessment, Appeal, and Regular Review

Either by self-application or referral from the care providers to their local government offices, potential service users must be screened and assessed by the standardized questionnaire. The questionnaire of 85 items is made up of 73 items covering 73 ADL items and 12 items covering mental ability and indicating dementia. The items were based on the study of time taken for service delivery in nursing homes rather than in home settings in the community. The questionnaire is administered by Care Managers who are either municipal officials or their commissioned professional representatives.

Following computerized analysis of the responses to these items, the results and doctor's letter are assessed by the local LTCI Assessment Committee for final ranking. In this way, individuals are classified as certified or not certified users, and the Care Rank of certified users and the amount of funding are determined. Funding is available for the full range of scheduled community services as detailed below, and for residential care, but if services beyond these are required, the client or the family must pay. Qualified Care Managers and the family of the aged individual are also involved in determining the Care Plan. A Care Rank registry is kept by the local municipalities for regular review, usually every six months.

If the individual and his or her family are not satisfied with the assessment outcome, they can initiate a second assessment, which is more clinically oriented, mostly with certification from medical doctors, and the case will be considered by the LTCI Assessment Council set up in each municipality in accordance with rules in Chapter 12 of the LTCI Law. The Assessment Council is made up of three by three by three membership appointed from the representatives of the insured, the municipality, and the public (Ishida & Sumii, 1999; Koseisho, 1999b; Yamamoto, 1999).

Scheduled Service Types

There are two major classes of scheduled LTCI services, one for the mostly home-based users and another for the institution-residential care users. The kinds of services at each Care Rank are set out in Table 1. The 12 types of services for the mostly home and mobile care cover visiting care (home help, bathing, nursing care, rehabilitation), mobile care at a day center, facility, or mobile rehabilitation, and care equipment rental, home care management consultation, short-stay nursing care or respite care, dementia type nursing care, and a special allowance for redesigning and upgrading the home infrastructure.

The three service types for residential care are Homes for the Elderly, which provide residential services for those who need a home because of social/familial difficulties; Special Aged Homes, which provide home services for those who have minor physical and/or mental problems but who could not be cared for by their families; and paramedical and clinically-based residential institutions, which provide residential nursing and allied health services for those who have more severe mental and physical health problems and who could not be cared for by their families. These institutions are now the most equivalent to nursing homes in other countries.

WILL THE EXPECTED OUTCOMES OF THE LTCI SCHEME BE ACHIEVED?

Notwithstanding six years of planning and preparation by the Ministry of Health and Welfare, the start of the LTCI scheme was belated, and some confusion arose because of the discrepancies between planning and reality. A number of points of contention arose over the period of the development of the LTCI scheme, and especially in the year immediately prior to the planned implementation. The rhetoric of much of the debate over these issues reflects the sparring relationship that exists in Japan between the bureaucracy on the one hand and service providers, professional practitioners, and academics on the other. Issues that the latter groups saw as threats to the integrity of the public welfare system were seen by the bureaucracy as opportunities for liberalizing the system. The following review of some of the problems identified by welfare professionals in the course of implementation demonstrates the tone of this debate.

The Public Welfare System Under Threat

The first and major issue concerned the adequacy of service provision that would be realized, and widespread shortfalls were cited. Of the services supposed to be available nationwide by April 2000, the levels actually available were 84% for home help, 72% for day services, and 76% for short-stay care. In about 10% of all municipalities, some 350 cities, towns, and villages, only half the planned level of home help was available, and 30% of municipalities could supply only 50% or less of visiting nurse services. Service providers also pointed out that while it had been envisaged that all eligible clients would have been assessed prior to the commencement of the scheme, by the end of February 2000, just one month before the LTCI scheme started, only around 1.17 million out of the 2.8 million eligible elderly had been assessed and given a defined Care Rank.

Service quality was a second widely debated issue. The prospect of private sector providers entering the field gave added force to this debate because no quality control mechanism had been put in place to cover this newly emerging sector. The lack of quality control was also raised as a problem in accreditation of Care Managers. Professionals made allegations that almost anyone could be accredited, and the level of knowledge required to pass the accreditation test would not require professional training. A particular contradiction was also seen in the potential for conflict of interest, as most Care Managers who had to make fair and independent Care Plans were actually employed by the service providers. Without a monitoring framework and quality control mechanism in place, the claims that the LTCI scheme would guarantee better services were derided as mere rhetoric.

Third, numerous aspects of the content and computerized processing of the schedule to be used in assessing care needs came under attack. Many of the points of criticism were similar to those raised with other assessment tools and processes, and include the reliability of assessments involving only single home visits; the way in which the role of family members was, or was not, to be taken into account; and the extent of detail, or lack of it, in the specification of criteria for independent performance of ADL vis-à-vis reliance on Care Managers' judgment. Dementia in particular was not seen to be fairly covered in the assessment. Professionals, objecting to what they saw as an overly quantitative approach to assessment, seized upon errors and anomalies in the piloting of the computer program.

Funding arrangements were a fourth area of contention. Variations in the tax base among municipalities, and hence in capacity to contribute to the LTCI scheme, loomed large, while the effectiveness of the national government's contribution to equalizing these variations remained untested. Concerns were also expressed about the capacity of users to meet the premiums and co-payments, and that municipalities would be left to pick up the difference.

Last of all, it was claimed that the level of service provided did not amount to effective support for home care and that the actual costs of caring for many elderly who were already receiving welfare services would exceed the funding provided under the insurance scheme. The new scheme was seen as being able to cover only a basic level of support and not promote quality of life more widely, with predictions of negative consequences for the elderly service recipients. The lack of provision of mental health services under the LTCI scheme came under particular attack.

These specific criticisms expressed the more general concern that the scheme was not welfare oriented and appeared to have been designed by people unfamiliar with welfare practice. Rather, bureaucrats were seen as intent on designing a sales mechanism that shuffled the elderly into one of the various emerging elderly care businesses, which were to provide a new haven for retiring bureaucrats just as the consumer finance sector had in the 1980s, resulting in new corporate-sector care providers under management that had no background experience in or orientation to welfare practice.

This debate added to the sense of insecurity about the new system, not just for the aged population, but also on the part of those responsible at the municipal level. According to a nation-wide survey conducted by Asahi Shimbun (November 24, 1999), 87% of municipal officials responsible for the LTCI scheme expressed some feelings of insecurity. Other studies suggested that most of the elderly who were aware of the new scheme felt more anxiety than about the previous health and welfare systems (Ambo, Lai, & Watanabe, 2000).

Not all the problems, whether predicted or newly emerging, had been ironed out prior to implementation. With services still in short supply, the government's efforts to explain how the delivery system would work were inadequate and increased pressure on providers and their staff, compounding uncertainty and feelings of unease among the aged and their families (Ambo, Lai, & Watanabe, 2000). Welfare professionals pointed out that the contracts between service providers and receivers being introduced with the new system were alien to Japanese society, especially for the culture of ordinary older citizens and their aging families. They went on to emphasize that with no experience of such contracts, neither the service providers nor the recipients had an understanding of what a good contract was, and further, that limitations of the Japanese legal system meant contracts could give only a nominal guarantee of service, not an enforceable one.

Liberalizing Long-Term Care

From the perspective of the central government, the new LTCI scheme changed the relationships among the aged, care providers, and the municipalities. Under the old system, municipalities commissioned the service providers to supply services directly to the aged clients. Under the LTCI scheme, there are now effectively three levels of contractual relationships. At the first level, the municipalities act as an insurance agency, and the aged clients have become the customers of this insurance agency; this relationship is public. A second level of contractual relationship has developed between the municipalities and the providers, through agreements that are conditional upon the terms of payment offered by the municipality, acting as the insurance agency, with reference to the status of the certified level of care need of the insured; it is not yet clear whether this relationship is fully public and open to scrutiny, or protected on grounds of being commercial-in-confidence. Third, the relationship between the insured client and the service providers is private in nature, though subject to the protection of the LTCI Law; this relationship is the area of greatest change.

The dual contractual arrangements between providers and municipalities on the one hand and providers and clients on the other open up the possibility for the providers, whether non-profit or profit-making, to invest and provide care services, resulting in long-term care becoming a more privatized service. At the very least, the private contractual relationships enable negotiation of terms of service beyond the standardized items, such as time and number of services provided.

Other aspects of the LTCI scheme reflect some of the basic features of public management via contractual agreements and a pro-market approach that characterize health care reform in Japan more widely. These features include the standardization of costing and pricing as exercised through the LTCI scheme; the division between policy development at the level of the central Ministry of Health and Welfare and implementation through municipalities and local service providers; the split of the municipalities' role as service purchasers from the provider role of private and non-profit agencies; and the widening of the choices available to individual households. All of these developments are intended to have a positive effect on stimulating a competitive, internal long-term care market. More importantly, they will have a significant impact on the promotion of long-term care as an industry, with a business-like mode of operation.

To prevent care providers from supplying the insured with more care services than they truly need, including unnecessarily long treatment, and hence charging more, the LTCI scheme has a built-in screening and review process for the certified category of service that specifies the entitlements and cost/price. All of these mechanisms have prepared a level playing field for profit-making agencies to enter the business of long-term care.

Initial estimates suggest that the new long-term care market will have a turnover of over ¥5 trillion when the LTCI scheme starts. While most existing providers are in the well-established, non-profit sector, many large corporations in the private service sector have expressed interest in the business of providing more cost-effective long-term care services for the insured. The increase in the number of registered service providers by April 2000 points to the possibility of further liberalization, if not commercialization, of the long-term care sector. At the same time as the LTCI Law has made provisions for service standards and quality control for the expanding long-term care industry, it remains to be seen how well it can protect the insured aged who are contracted customers of the providers (*Kaigohoken Monthly,* June 2000, No. 52).

A CONTINUING DEBATE

The LTCI scheme represents a kind of safety net of which the public can take full advantage. Although it still leaves much to be desired, the scheme is vital to the struggle to meet the challenges posed by the aging of the population in the future. At a macro level, the LTCI scheme should have a demonstrative effect for reforms in social security and taxation that are in the pipeline, and the provision of a safety net for long-term care should regain some of the community's trust in the administrative-political system.

Although some aspects of the LTCI scheme have been controversial, the scheme is seen as one step for coping with the problems of the bedridden elderly especially, and more importantly, as it has given increased impetus to rehabilitation for the elderly, thus reducing the number who are bedridden. By doing so, it is certain not only to help give elderly clients a sense of purpose, but also to relieve the strain on the depleted coffers of the health insurance system. At the household and family level, the LTCI scheme should deliver a better alternative than the previous arrangements, with professionally guided Care Plans for aging kin, notwithstanding the possible increase of insurance contributions and the cost effects on household income.

How the Care Plans will work through the whole system, for the benefit of the elderly and their households, remains to be seen. But at the very least, there seem to be open channels and systematic mechanisms for addressing the "hidden" social costs of caring for the aged, such as the uneven burden carried by women. The difficulties faced by individual households in caring (or not caring) for the aged have now been put into the public discourse and are on the public policy agenda. For this reason alone, the LTCI scheme will open up a new era of debate on aging in Japanese society in the 21st century.

REFERENCES

Ambo, N., Watanabe, R., & Lai, On-Kwok (2000). *Research Report on Nursing Care Insurance in the Higashi Harima (Hyogo Prefecture).* Kagogawa City: Federation of the Nursing Homes for the Aged in Higashi Harima Area.

Asahi, K. (1999). *Kaigohoken no Point* [Points of Long-Term Care Insurance]. Tokyo: Kiri Shobo.

Hiramatsu, K. (1999). *Kagohoken Service* [Long-Term Care Service]. Tokyo: Dental-Medico-Pharmaceutical Publishers.

Ishida, K., & Sumii, H. (1999). *Kaigohoken-Assessment* [Long-Term Care Insurance Assessment]. Tokyo: Hubunsha.

Ito, S. (1997). *Kaigohoken* [Long-Term Care Insurance]. Tokyo: Aoki-Shoten.

Kaigohoken Monthly (Long-Term Care Insurance Monthly), June 2000, No. 52.

Komuro, A., & Nagatani, N. (1999*). Kaigohoken, Shakkai Fukushi pou* [Long-Term Care, Social Welfare Laws]. Tokyo: Bookman-sha.

Koseisho [Ministry of Health & Welfare]. (1999a). *Kosei [Health & Welfare] White Paper.* Tokyo: Koseisho.

Koseisho [Ministry of Health & Welfare]. (1999b). *Shakkai Fukushi no Direction* [Direction of Social Welfare]. Tokyo: Koseisho.

Matsui, S. (1999). *Nihonkoku kempou* [Japanese Constitution]. Tokyo: Yuhi-kaku.

Minerva, S. (1999). *Shakkai Fukuishi Shoropou* [Six Laws on Social Welfare]. Tokyo: Minerva Shobou.

Yamamoto, K. (1999). *Kaigohoken & Rehabilitation* [Long Term Care and Rehabilitation].Tokyo: Kosei Science Institute.

Zenkoku Rojin Fukushi Kyogikai [ZRFK] (1999). *Hokatsuteki jiritsu shien Program–Kaigo Service Keikaku Sakusei Manual* [Manual and Service Programming for Independent Living]. Tokyo: Shakai Fukushi Pouren ZRFK.

Long-Term Care Policy and Financing as a Public or Private Matter in the United States

Donna L. Yee, PhD

Executive Director, Asian Community Center,
Sacramento, California

SUMMARY. Effective approaches to assure adequate resources, infrastructure, and broad societal support to address chronic care needs are volatile and potentially unpopular issues that can result in many losers (those getting far less than they want) and few winners (those who gain access to scarce societal resources for care). In the United States, debates on long-term care involve a complex set of issues and services that link health, social services (welfare), and economic policies that often pit public and private sector interests and values against one another. Yet long-term care policies fill a necessary function in society to clarify roles, expectations, and functions of public, non-profit, for profit, indi-

---

Dr. Donna L. Yee received her PhD in Social Policy from the Heller School at Brandeis University in 1990. She is Executive Director of the Asian Community Center in Sacramento, CA. Her studies are related to health and long-term care policy, service access, quality of care and other issues affecting older Asian and Pacific Islander persons in the United States. Dr. Yee has 25 years of experience in long-term care. Her health administration and clinical experience (14 years) includes work at an 1100-bed public chronic care facility, On Lok Senior Health Services, and at a home health agency.

Dr. Yee can be contacted at the Asian Community Center, 7801 Rush River Drive, Sacramento, CA 95831, USA (E-mail: dly346@juno.com).

[Haworth co-indexing entry note]: "Long-Term Care Policy and Financing as a Public or Private Matter in the United States." Yee, Donna L. Co-published simultaneously in *Journal of Aging & Social Policy* (The Haworth Press, Inc.) Vol. 13, No. 2/3, 2001, pp. 35-51; and: *Long-Term Care in the 21st Century: Perspectives from Around the Asia-Pacific Rim* (ed: Iris Chi, Kalyani K. Mehta, and Anna L. Howe) The Haworth Press, Inc., 2001, pp. 35-51. Single or multiple copies of this article are available for a fee from The Haworth Document Delivery Service [1-800-HAWORTH, 9:00 a.m. - 5:00 p.m. (EST). E-mail address: getinfo@haworthpressinc.com].

35

vidual, and family sectors of a society. By assessing and developing policy proposals that include all long-term care system dimensions, a society can arrive at systematic, fair, and rational decisions. Limiting decisions to system financing aspects alone is likely to result in unforeseen or unintended effects in a long-term care system that stopgap "fixes" cannot resolve. Three underlying policy challenges are presented: the need for policymakers to consider whether the public sector is the first or last source of payment for long-term care; whether government is seen primarily as a risk or cost manager; and the extent to which choice is afforded to elders and family caregivers with regard to the types, settings, and amount of long-term care desired to complement family care. *[Article copies available for a fee from The Haworth Document Delivery Service: 1-800-HAWORTH. E-mail address: <getinfo@haworthpressinc.com> Website: <http://www.HaworthPress.com> © 2001 by The Haworth Press, Inc. All rights reserved.]*

KEYWORDS. Long-term care financing, long-term care insurance, private/public roles

POLICY CONTEXT AND OBJECTIVES

The need to focus on the chronic care needs of large numbers of older adults has been a topic of national debate since late in the 20th century in the United States, and it continues to compete for its place on the policy agenda into the first decade of the 21st century. Advances in public health and medical science in conjunction with growing stability among social, economic, and political conditions in nations and global regions have contributed to significant longevity gains. As populations and individuals begin to raise concerns about the desired quality of life in a person's later years and related demands on society to meet increasing amounts and kinds of long-term social and health care needs, policymakers are challenged to address the social, financial, and sometimes political impacts of increasing numbers and proportions of older adults in their jurisdictions.

Policy efforts in long-term care in the United States can be grouped on the basis of three broad objectives: those aiming to (1) lower the incidence of chronic care needs, (2) manage, ration, and minimize outlays of both financial and human resources to mediate chronic care needs, and (3) emphasize family or informal caregiving as the preferred, most responsive, and least costly source of chronic care.

First, policies to lower the incidence of chronic care needs among all sectors of the population have used public health campaigns to promote healthy lifestyles, prevent disease, and broadly present health as the absence of disease. National efforts have focused on individual and community interventions. As well, private health care insurance programs have attempted to identify incentives to promote individual fitness and healthy lifestyle habits. And finally, the newest benefits in the largest United States insurance program, Medicare, include services to detect disease processes early and impress on individuals the desirability of early treatment.

Second, policies using financing mechanisms to achieve efficient use of financial and human resources to deliver chronic care have been the more visible aspects of debates about chronic care or long-term care in the United States (Kingson, 1996). Concern in several states that nursing home costs alone could unbalance government budgets if not managed or curbed prompted state initiatives that have relocated individuals from nursing homes to home, community-based, or residential programs. Distinctions between "skilled" and "custodial" types of chronic care have a large impact on public and insurance funds available to pay for care. A system historically driven by hospital and acute medical care, whose primary purpose is measured improvement in health status and functioning, has often failed to address the medical needs among the increasing numbers of people living longer with one or more chronic conditions that lead to disability. This approach poorly addresses the nature of chronic care needs, and it results in missed opportunities to avoid some of the high costs of care.

Third, policies that guard public expenditure from becoming a replacement for family care have been visible as part of explicit discussions on public versus private long-term care obligations among family members for two decades and longer (Binstock, 1998). Studies in the United States consistently suggest that formal services enable family caregivers to sustain their caregiving efforts by providing respite and recognizing that it is often unrealistic to expect family members to provide increasing amounts of care as family members become frailer. No study has found that provision of skilled and home-based support services led family caregivers to neglect or abandon their elders. Employer and public interests in assuring the availability of adult sons and daughters to work and optimize their productivity often play a factor in enabling many informal caregivers to choose employment in addition to coordinating care schedules and tasks with formal services.

Policymakers and analysts who raise these issues and press for more effective approaches to assure that countries will have resources, infrastructure, and broad societal support for addressing chronic care needs are showing an unusual courage. These are volatile and potentially unpopular public policy issues that result in many losers (those getting far less than they want) and few winners (those who gain access to scarce societal resources for care). In the United States, debates about long-term care often involve a complex set of issues and services that overlap and link with health, social services (welfare), and even economic policies. To capture the tone and scope of this debate in the United States, this paper presents an overall framework within which specific aspects of long-term care policy in the United States can be highlighted.

PRINCIPLES AND PHILOSOPHY OF THE UNITED STATES' LONG-TERM CARE FRAMEWORK

Long-term care policy refers to decisions at national, local, and administrative levels (public and private) that set the ground rules that define, finance, organize, deliver, and manage long-term care systems. Drawing on the work of Capitman (1990) and the Institute for Health Policy at Brandeis University (1992), an analytic framework for long-term care policy discussions in the United States and many other countries can be set out in five system dimensions as follows.

Long-Term Care System Goals and Their Underlying Values

Long-term care system goals and their underlying values are important to consider because long-term care systems reflect the ways in which a society highly values, is neutral to, or ostracizes its most frail aged members and those with physical disability (Cowart, 1996; Daniels, 1998). If a government wants to assure optimal productivity among all workers, it might provide care for children and adults who are not adequately productive in the work force. Services for the dependent (those with physical or emotional disability) might be made available so that economic productivity of those who would otherwise provide care to them would not be hampered. Alternatively, if a government believes that the head of each family has responsibility for the welfare of family members, there would be little government intervention and families would rely on their own members or (in a market economy) pay for care they do not provide themselves. Additionally, if a government believes that market forces, including employers (corporations), should determine when and whether it is in their best interest to provide charitable care for children and infirm older persons, then government might assume small gap-filling roles to meet residents' community-level long-term care needs that are not met by family members or businesses.

Whether a system punishes or compassionately supports those needing long-term care, society's values and goals are reflected in its long-term care policies. Long-term care policies give shape to those goals and values by indicating the levels and types of responsibilities and roles that are portioned to government, community structures, family members, and individuals. By extension, long-term care policies indicate the extent to which long-term care is seen as a public or private responsibility. The good news is that not everyone in a society will need long-term care. The bad news is that no one knows which individuals among us will need long-term care.

Benefit Structure

A benefit structure is an array of services or programs for providing long-term care. Services such as homemaker care, adult day health care, transportation assistance, home-delivered meals, residential care, nursing home (skilled nursing facility care), and others are available in many countries as well as in the United States. Decisions to include or exclude different services often reflect service approaches that are culturally acceptable and consistent with a society's goals and norms. For example, services that emphasize care in the home might focus on assistance with instrumental tasks rather than socialization, and care in a group setting might emphasize rehabilitation rather than custodial care. Socialization and custodial care may be seen as less important and a less effective use of scarce dollars, compared to assistance with instrumental tasks that support independence, and rehabilitation that improves functioning.

Organization of Service Delivery

Organization of service delivery refers to the way services are or are not connected to one another. Delivery systems reflect whether continuity of care is valued across levels of care and/or among specialized services. As well, referral patterns and eligibility rules determine how service resources are distributed or rationed among those needing care. Service delivery systems implement long-term care policies that set expectations for which services are available, accessible, and affordable to people according to their types of long-term care needs. As well, service delivery systems can influence the types and mix of service providers and their performance or standards for quality care. Delivery systems are the ways in which benefits have an order.

Third-Party and User Financing

Financing is related to who pays for what, when, and how. In the United States much of the payment for acute and medical care is through "third parties," whereby individuals largely rely on insurance mechanisms rather than out-of-pocket payments (between the buyer and seller of care) when a service is used. The insurer becomes a "third party" that increasingly intervenes in what the buyer and seller of a service arrange. While many see this as a disadvantage because it blocks direct negotiations and accountability between the patient and the expert helper, in the United States, for example, insurance schemes have the financing advantage of minimizing individual risks for care costs so that care becomes affordable. Alternately, non-acute medical and other costs of chronic care are not generally insured in the United States. Impoverishment from the costs of long-term care over time has become an increasingly predictable risk as older persons live longer with chronic care needs. The low proportion of elders receiving any long-term care services at any one time belies the much higher risk of needing some support over any individual's whole lifetime.

As costs for long-term care and numbers of older persons with chronic care needs increase, insurance programs may be a reliable mechanism to pool funds contributed by a large number of people so that costs of care can be affordable among them. Long-term care financing policy in the United States reflects changes in expectations of how government or individual families will meet long-term care needs and costs. Government social insurance programs have an interest in efficiently "covering" all people with needs, by making benefits available only to those who meet certain criteria.

Early versions of the Older Americans Act state that all persons 60 and older who need help with everyday activities due to health problems could be eligible for a range of care services funded under that law. Complementary social welfare laws paid for other services needed by the poor, such as housekeeping, laundry, shopping, personal care, and transportation to medical appointments.

Concern with the growing costs of these programs resulted in policies to limit program benefits, funding, eligibility for services, or service availability. Some efforts set predetermined limits on outlays for the amount and kind of service use per person per month. Other approaches used rules to limit the number of persons eligible for programs. Still others require consumers to pay larger shares of service costs based on their incomes. Methods to curb costs and manage outlays rarely responded to the needs for long-term care within communities, but they continue as common rationing methods. In the United States, among those with personal wealth, individuals are expected to purchase whatever services they need and can afford in the market, but market failure due to lack of workers, poor care, and lack of appropriate service settings often means that even money cannot buy a person the long-term care he or she needs.

Private long-term care insurance products are increasingly available to insure for nursing home care, primarily, and home health care to a lesser degree.

Costs are high and benefits generally do not cover the more common situations in which long-term care is needed. These products have yet to be affordable and responsive to the risks consumers face for a range of long-term care needs (Lieberman, 1995; Weiner, 1996). As a result, there are almost as many proponents for further development of private financing products as for public financing programs. Furthermore, long-term care needs, use, and costs across a diverse U. S. population increase the difficulty of defining an insurance product and testing its feasibility (Yee, 1998).

System Administration

Finally, the system administration dimension of long-term care systems in the public sector has more recently begun to monitor and synthesize information on the use of system benefits, service delivery, financing, and whether or not the system is achieving its goals. In some administrative structures, case managers have responsibility for assessing consumer needs, determining eligibility for specific types of long-term care services, coordinating/acquiring needed services, and monitoring individual service plans. In the United States, administrative case management occurs most often in government or other insurance programs that oversee outlays for care and control individual access to institutional (high cost) services. Independent private practice case managers, alternatively, are often advocates who negotiate on behalf of the consumer to acquire needed help.

Long-term care policies in the United States fill a necessary function in society to clarify roles, expectations, and functions of public, non-profit, for profit, individual, and family sectors of a society. By assessing and developing policy proposals that include all long-term care system dimensions, a society can arrive at systematic, fair, and rational decisions. Limiting decisions to system financing aspects alone is likely to result in unforeseen or unintended effects in a long-term care system that stopgap "fixes" cannot resolve. This problem is especially apparent in the United States where health care and long-term care policies intersect.

PROBLEMS GENERATED BY LACK OF A LONG-TERM CARE POLICY

The lack of an explicit national long-term care policy has become an increasing challenge in the United States since Medicare was established as a major federal health insurance program for older adults, and Medicaid as a parallel program for the poor, in 1965. Most long-term care policymaking remains at the state and local government levels. It is difficult to address systematically long-term care or chronic care needs of a growing number of older adults in every community on a national basis. Instead, a "problem-generated long-term care policy" ensues, as four examples illustrate.

Poor Quality Care

The United States has an array of "entrepreneurial" programs reflecting different ideas and goals that sometimes conflict. Some policies treat health and long-term care as a "public" good and some as a "private" good. Many policies in the United States imply that individual health and long-term care needs can be adequately met by free market forces. As a result, some parts of long-term care service delivery finance profit-takers who provide poor care: These are service providers more interested in paying shareholders short-term returns on investment than in caring for frail older persons, especially those who are poor. This situation occurs in all sectors of the nursing home, home health agency, and assisted living/residential care industry in the United States.

One set of policy responses has been by way of a number of "consumer protection" laws and regulations that do not change service delivery, but set expectations and (some would say) mild sanctions for performance among service providers. A limitation of these approaches is that an older person or family member must initiate a complaint against the provider before an investigation is launched. The investigation does not guarantee a solution that improves care or stops an abuse. Family and whistleblower concerns about retaliation and ostracism are a strong disincentive to get the benefits of consumer protections.

Recent visible efforts in the United States have sought to assure that, as a "consumer" of services or an insurance program "beneficiary," the individual and family members are afforded choices about when care is provided (e.g., every day or two days per week), the setting of care (e.g., home care versus adult day center care), and which agency is designated as provider of care. Notions of consumer-driven care, including programs where poor consumers are given cash to purchase their choice of services, have gained credence in the last five years. As components of the long-term care service system become increasingly proprietary, consumer choices are considered a prevailing curb on "market" excesses (Capitman & Sciegaj, 1995; Hall et al., 1994; Hibbard & Jewett, 1996; Leutz et al., 1988a; Yee et al., 1999).

Whether a long-term care service is funded by public or private sources, consumer-driven approaches hold that frail elders and their family members can get enough information about available services and different service providers to reach decisions that are the best value for their dollar. Further, "markets" will support competition among providers so that worries about whether care is of adequate quality can be controlled by the market rather than regulated by the government. Some policymakers in the United States believe that when trade-offs among quality, availability, and price are made by consumers, they share the risk of acquiring appropriate, affordable, and accessible care. Others believe that relying on a "market" driven long-term care system of supply and demand puts unrealistic burdens on the consumer (and family members) because access to enough information and choices among affordable providers of high-quality, "need-driven" care places consumers in a vulnerable rather than a strong negotiating position.

Most consumers and advocates in the United States would not credit "market approaches" with assuring that adequate care standards are met among long-term care service providers. There is persisting uncertainty in at least three areas: whether decisions to get care "A" or care "B" represent the best balanced response to clinical and financial needs; fear that needed care cannot be acquired in a timely manner, even when relying on expert gatekeepers such as case managers to get the right care; and a sense of vulnerability because little is known about how to assure that care outcomes can be associated with consumer decisions and expectations. In the United States, many older persons still rely on family doctors or expert case managers in making decisions, and few people plan ahead and feel knowledgeable and ready to make long-term care and geriatric care decisions. An effort to make the best coerced decision based on expert input, assuming those experts are in fact widely knowledgeable, is the norm. Making a consumer choice model work effectively in the United States is still largely a work in progress, even as it is a cornerstone for current efforts to assure quality care and optimize cost and benefits for persons needing chronic care.

Controlling Escalation of Long-Term Care Costs

Reform efforts increasingly in the last 25 years rely on policies to address uncontrolled growth in public and individual outlays for long-term care. In the 1980s, fear that nursing home costs would consume the Medicaid program resulted in regulations and laws to limit severely the expansion or new construction of nursing homes, to direct portions of reimbursement rates toward wages of the lowest paid nursing assistants rather than shareholders, and to increase the number of direct-care staff required in nursing homes. Concurrently, many advocates and policymakers in local communities put pressure on state governments to increase funds for home and community-based long-term care services.

Other initiatives aimed to control costs have seen a narrowing of coverage of long-term care programs, with a concentration on skilled nursing services. Increased waiting lists and program regulations serve to ration access to services, and the common administrative response appears to have been to give more older persons "some" care, while not knowing whether the care received is adequate for their needs (Leutz et al., 1988b; Shaughnessy & Kramer, 1990; Vladeck, Miller, & Clauser, 1993; Weiner, Stevenson, & Goldenson, 1998).

As the average age of those in the United States rises, it can be expected that greater numbers of persons will be familiar with institutional and community-based long-term care service systems. It is possible that efforts to control long-term care costs as a proportion of health or other social service outlays will continue to rely on politically acceptable mechanisms that narrowly target (ration) access to publicly funded long-term care services. Perhaps, in the political context in the United States, a benefit is that constituencies that vote can get targeting criteria modified to benefit different groups of people without substantially increasing their outlays. In this scenario there will always be sectors of the population who do not get the long-term care help they need. The challenge, though, is that unless larger numbers of older adults remain "healthy" and disability-free into their later years, small policy adjustments will not address the potential demand for long-term care in the United States from 2020 onward.

Long-Term Care System Fragmentation

The third example of "problem-generated policy" stems from problems among elders in getting a concerted mix of long-term care services when most needed. Poor continuity of care continues to be a reason for avoidable hospitalizations, falls, and instances of neglect among elders in the service system. More explicit rules were initiated to define how, when, and where patients could use Medicare nursing home benefits or home health benefits upon discharge from an acute hospital in order to assure that the most frail received care they need. In these instances case managers must implement targeting policies by helping the patient/consumer navigate different service systems to get the best value for public dollars spent on services. A benefit of such targeting approaches is that those who are most frail get needed assistance. The less frail, while admittedly needing care, however, might not get any assistance. By reducing costs of care for those who are likely to be the most costly cases overall, policies developed to target that group resulted in a lower likelihood for those less frail and in stable situations to get care they needed (Branch & Stuart, 1984; Leutz et al., 1992; Weissert, 1985).

Among the most successful program linkage demonstrations aimed at improving continuity of care have been initiatives that evolved from pilot projects with government and charitable foundation funding over the last 25 years. These long-term care policy experiments tested ideas to broaden the benefit package offered to consumers by (a) integrating Medicare, Medicaid, and Older Americans Act benefits in ways that overcame service barriers and inefficiencies caused by maintaining segregated program records and access for each program, (b) changing service delivery by funneling service acquisition and access through one provider that also managed service organization and financial relationships, and (c) sharing financial risks for the cost of care among insuring (government programs) and service providers (Ansak, 1990; Branch, Coulam, & Zimmerman, 1995). One demonstration project that became a national program is detailed in the next article, "The Program of All-Inclusive Care for the Elderly (PACE): An Innovative Long-Term Care Model in the United States."

Social Health Maintenance Organizations (SHMOs) were a second demonstration concurrently operated in community hospitals or health maintenance organizations. They modeled ways of managing chronic care needs and negotiating care arrangements among providers, and offer consumers a budget for their service choices to achieve lower costs and increased cost control while assuring high-quality care focused on individual optimal functioning and independence (Leutz et al., 1988b; Vladeck et al., 1993).

Among many policy analysts, these demonstrations and integration efforts among acute medical, hospital, and long-term care costs, and service delivery provide the most useful models for assuring (a) continuity among services in these settings that enhances outcomes for those with multiple chronic health problems, (b) adequate control and flexibility in the organization of services, and (c) shared risk and responsibility for cost control and management among the insurer, consumer, and service provider.

Long-Term Care Defined by System Boundaries

The absence of an explicit, overall national long-term care policy in the United States has resulted in a long-term care system defined by the boundaries of other systems. The long-term care system in the United States is actually a "residual" of other health and social service systems, with "residual" meaning what is left over after the "best" parts are consumed. Long-term care is a residual set of services and client needs that do not get paid for by other explicitly defined service systems, partly because of fear of the unknown "risks of occurrence" or how often people might need or use long-term care.

A relatively recent example of "residualization" in the United States is the emergence of "sub-acute" care, which straddles the long-term care and acute care systems. Policies to reduce drastically acute hospital costs under Medicare and Medicaid established payments based on the average cost of a stay for specific conditions and necessary treatments, thereby closing an existing open-ended source of funds for providers. Payment for Diagnostic Related Groups placed hospitals at risk for unjustified long stays and hospital readmissions, which implies poor care was provided. Older patients were discharged "sicker and quicker" so that hospitals would not be caught with costs for which they could not get payment. Nursing homes, however, were generally unable to take patients needing complex, technical, and intensive skilled nursing care. A new level of sub-acute care emerged, more intense than nursing home care, but less complex than acute hospital care. Government did not reduce expenditures through this policy by as much as they hoped. Some of the reductions were expended on sub-acute care for patients rescued from situations where they needed care and there was no willing service provider.

From 1987 to 1994, Medicare and Medicaid outlays in the United States increased overall by 25% (in constant 1994 dollars), but there is a sharp difference between the earlier and later years. Between 1987 and 1990, the increase was only 7%, largely due to "savings" in acute hospital outlays as a result of the policies that (a) drastically reduced stays of older persons in acute hospitals, (b) limited the supply of nursing home beds, and (c) encouraged the growth of home health agency services. As a result, outlays for nursing home and home health care increased, and in the period 1990 to 1994, total outlays increased by 17%. Increases in nursing home and home health care were accommodated by controlling outlays for acute hospital and physician care (previously the highest expense categories). At the same time, aggressive efforts in many communities to expand non-institutional home- and community-based care services were also funded by reducing services for "well" elders. Most analysts conclude that policies to restrain costs in ways that targeted specific parts of the health care system successfully avoided otherwise expected increases of 20% or more in outlays (HCFA, 1996).

One impact of controlling outlays on hospital and physician care was a higher demand for technical and intensive nursing for frail elders at home. Several pilot programs tested "downward delegation" of what had been defined as skilled nursing or physician levels of care. These policies allow lower-level professionals or paraprofessionals to do specified "medical" or "nursing" tasks under supervision. One outcome has been an increased demand for mid-level practitioners such as nurse practitioners, geriatric specialist nurses, or physician assistants, who manage specified types of chronic diseases. Downward delegation addresses shortages among (more costly) primary care physicians in some communities and care settings, while supporting mid-level practitioners (less costly) who also use a greater array of low-tech interventions, such as spending more time with the patient, visiting more frequently, and supervising caregivers to assure treatment compliance that highly trained physician specialists are less inclined to carry out.

POLICY CHALLENGES

In the United States, many decisions about long-term care are driven as much by the search for solutions to financing problems as by a shared sense of the societal goals, values, and mission. As in other countries, many in the United States try to balance financing decisions about long-term care with a shared sense of "goals, values, and mission" because we believe that such an approach would assure a humane, cost-effective, and rational long-term care system that responds to diverse consumer preferences. A part of this discussion has been an effort to understand better societal expectations about public and private roles in financing long-term care (Walker, Bradley, & Wetle, 1998). The dichotomy of public and private roles seems simple, but it underestimates the diversity of the non-government sector in the United States, which includes non-profit, for profit, and family/individual perspectives.

In the United States, there is a stronger emphasis on the individual as a consumer than on the shared values of families or communities when roles and responsibilities for meeting health care needs are considered. These roles and responsibilities broadly include knowing which services are available to meet particular needs, paying for them, and making choices or selections among formal and informal care options. In a system that is driven by "private" interests, individuals with some ability to pay for a portion of their own care (but little wealth) are the most vulnerable because they are more likely to get inadequate amounts of long-term care compared to either the poor (due to government safety net programs) or the wealthy. Those with some resources are more likely to be forced to choose between the needs of their children and their own needs, or between their current needs and the potential for larger, more costly needs as their frailty increases.

While many adult children continue to pay for parent care, this is largely limited to those families with enough wealth and income to address competing obligations such as college and education costs for grandchildren, personal savings for retirement, and a fading sense of financial obligation toward elder parents. As well, elders increasingly say they do not expect to ask adult children for assistance, preferring to apply to the government rather than be a burden on adult children (AARP, 2001). In this context, demand alone does not drive supply, because large numbers of the demanders (i.e., those needing long-term care) do not have adequate personal resources to get care. The government or another third party paying for care has a bigger impact on the market. Three policy challenges arise from differences in views regarding the role that government or other third parties should take.

First or Last Payer?

The first policy challenge is whether the government or public sector role is to be the First payer and prime policymaker, versus the Last payer and one of several policymakers. As first payer, government would be the prime policymaker, controlling and managing available financial and service delivery resources. An expectation might be that government should be innovative in assuring fair, efficient, and effective management of resources in order to ensure that those needing long-term care get the best care from the defined resource pool. As first payer, government can also become coercive, focused on system efficiency in ways that severely constrain consumer choice about what care is delivered, how, and in what setting.

As last payer, the government would be one of several stakeholders involved in long-term care policymaking. In this scenario, perhaps with non-profit organizations, businesses, and influential individuals, government's main role would be to emphasize the need for private-sector solutions that reach as many people as possible (in terms of service access, availability, acceptability, and affordability). In the United States, various elected administrators have taken different positions along this continuum, which has resulted in a mix of policies. Public-sector (federal, state, and local governments) roles and motivation to develop good long-term care policies differ greatly across communities in the United States. Policies responding to concern that an over-reliance on market forces may not provide adequate protection for the most vulnerable consumers have led to "patients' rights" or "consumer protection" regulations and rules. These policies aim to level the playing field between big business health institutions and chronically ill individuals with disability.

Risk or Cost Manager?

A second policy challenge is to consider the extent to which government's role is to be the manager of risks or costs in the long-term care system. The initial Medicaid law incorporated incentives to reimburse construction of nursing homes in the nursing home care rates. As costs of publicly financed long-term care between 1965 and 1975 escalated, policies were initiated to develop "al-

ternative" settings for long-term care that lowered cost and were more acceptable to families. In effect, funding for home- and community-based care was a
way of separating real estate costs from service delivery and benefit costs because individual clients remain at home. Increases in the number of frail older
adults, however, have resulted in greater system demands that require more
than the "savings" captured by policies to emphasize alternative, less costly
home- and community-based care.

Because long-term care costs continue to threaten to impoverish larger
numbers of older persons and their family members in the United States (the
cost for a one-year nursing home stay is about $50,000 US), there is a greater
incentive to expand financing and rationing mechanisms, even in the context
of variation across local community service systems. As a result, the United
States government has taken on broader roles as a risk manager: It monitors
costs of care among "levels of care" or types of need for care by using objective and reliable measures of physical and cognitive functioning that affect a
person's ability to sustain an independent living arrangement. Studies to link
reimbursement rates with the level (or amount) of care needed by individuals
or "case mix reimbursement" are underway and are part of efforts to determine
how to set "all inclusive" rates for defined subsets of care (e.g., Resource Utilization Groups in nursing homes, Prospective Payment System in home health
agencies, Capitation rates for Program for All Inclusive Services for the Elderly or PACE sites). These studies point to significant challenges in the
United States with regard to (a) gathering information that can support fair decisions for distributing access to benefits on a population basis, (b) accumulat-
ing knowledge so that the technology exists to identify those who have the
highest risks, and (c) assuring that appropriate interventions are available to
mediate risks. In these areas, after 35 years of effort, long-term care programs
in the United States are still struggling. Many of the differences in long-term
care availability reflect variation in rules about who should get scarce resources.

Choice for Elders and Family Caregivers?

A third set of policy challenges is to clarify parameters of "choice" for elders and their family caregivers. This area of concern is perhaps the most recent addition to policy discussions in the United States. For example, the new
Administration on Aging National Family Caregiver Support Program focuses
on helping community service systems respond to the diversity of caregiver
needs and ways to assure that choices will be available (see www.AoA.gov/
carenetwork). While "choice" is necessary in a theoretical free-market economy, policies that support the idea that "benefits" and "service organization

and delivery" should be responsive to varied individual and family preferences for care and situations, would result in some local variation in settings of care (i.e., institution, home, day center) as well as in goals for care (i.e., curative, palliative, restorative, and maintenance). Meetings to encourage explicit participation in determination of standards for the quantity, quality, and service delivery modes in a local area would involve consumers in assuring that services meet their goals and standards for care. Even while central government efforts to set standards for quality of care and to monitor quality are being developed in the United States, most providers and family caregivers know that, just as in schools for children, involvement of family caregivers and leaders in the community is what assures quality on a day-to-day basis in every long-term care setting.

REFERENCES

AARP (2001). *In the middle: A report on multicultural boomers coping with family and aging issues.* Washington, DC: AARP.

Ansak, M. L. (1990). On Lok model: Consolidating care and financing. *Generations, 14*(2): 73-74.

Binstock, R. H. (1998). The financing and organization of long-term care. In L. C. Walker, E. H. Bradley and T. Wetle (Eds.), *Public and private responsibilities in long-term care.* Baltimore: Johns Hopkins University Press: 1-24.

Branch, L., Coulam, R., & Zimmerman, Y. (1995). The PACE evaluation: Initial findings. *The Gerontologist, 35*(3): 349-359.

Branch, L. G., & Stuart, N. E. (1984). Five-year history of targeting home care services to prevent institutionalization. *The Gerontologist, 24*(4): 387-391.

Capitman, J. A. (1990). Policy and program options in community-oriented long-term care. In M. P. Lawton (Ed.), *Annual review of gerontology and geriatrics* (Vol. 9, 1989, pp. 357-388). New York, NY: Springer Publishing Company.

Capitman, J. A., & Sciegaj, M. (1995). A contextual approach for understanding individual autonomy in managed community long-term care. *The Gerontologist, 35*(4): 533-540.

Cowart, M. (1996). Long-term care policy and the American family. *Journal of Aging & Social Policy, 7*(3-4): 169-184.

Daniels, N. (1998). Justice and prudential deliberation in long-term care. In L. C. Walker, E. H. Bradley and T. Wetle (Eds.). *Public and private responsibilities in long-term care.* Baltimore: Johns Hopkins University Press: 93-114.

Hall, J. A., Irish, J. T., Roter, D. L., Ehrlich, C. M., & Miller, L. H. (1994). Satisfaction, gender, and communication in medical visits. *Medical Care, 32*(12): 1216-1231.

HCFA. (1996). *Health care financing REVIEW statistical supplement* (Pub No. 03386). Baltimore, MD: United States Department of Health and Human Services, Health Care Financing Administration, Office of Research and Demonstration.

Hibbard, J. H., & Jewett, J. J. (1996). What type of quality information do consumers want in a health care report card? *Medical Care Research and Review, 53*(1): 28-47.

Institute for Health Policy, Brandeis University (1992). *How healthy is your community care system? An eldercare assessment guide.* National Eldercare Institute on Long-Term Care, National Association of State Units on Aging, Washington, DC.

Kingson, E. (1996). Ways of thinking about the long-term care of the baby-boom cohorts. *Journal of Aging & Social Policy, 7*(3-4): 3-23.

Leutz, W., Capitman, J., MacAdam, M., & Abrahams, R. (1992). *Care for frail elders: Developing community solutions.* New York, NY: Auburn House.

Leutz, W., Capitman, J. A., Abrahams, R., Pendleton, S., & Omata, R. (1988a). *Strategies for strengthening long-term care: Issues, choices for America.* Institute for Health Policy, Brandeis University, Waltham, MA.

Leutz, W. N., Abrahams, R., Greenlick, M., Kane, R., & Prottas, J. (1988b). Targeting expanded care to the aged: Early SHMO experience. *Gerontologist, 28*(1): 4-17.

Lieberman, T. (1995). Who pays for the nursing home? *Consumer Reports, 60* (September): 591-597.

Shaughnessy, P. W., & Kramer, A. M. (1990). The increased needs of patients in nursing homes and patients receiving home health care. *The New England Journal of Medicine, 322*(1): 21-27.

Vladeck, B. C., Miller, N. A., & Clauser, S. B. (1993). The changing face of long-term care. *Health Care Financing Review, 14*(4): 5-23.

Walker, L. C., Bradley, E., & Wetle, T. (Eds.). (1998). *Public and private responsibilities in long-term care: Finding the balance.* Baltimore: Johns Hopkins University Press.

Weissert, W. (1985). Seven reasons why it is so difficult to make community-based long term care cost-effective. *Health Services Research, 20*(4): 423-433.

Wiener, J. (1996). Financing reform for long-term care: Strategies for public and private long-term care insurance. *Journal of Aging & Social Policy, 7*(3-4): 109-27.

Wiener, J. M., Stevenson, D. G., & Goldenson, S. M. (1998). *Controlling the supply of long-term care providers at the state level* (Occasional Paper No. 22). Washington, DC: The Urban Institute.

Yee, D. L. (1998). Community perceptions of public and private responsibility in the context of cultural diversity. In L. C. Walker, E. H. Bradley and T. Wetle (Eds.). *Public and private responsibilities in long-term care: Finding the balance.* Baltimore: Johns Hopkins University Press.

Yee, D. L., Capitman, J. A., Leutz, W. N., & Sciegaj, M. (1999). A resident-centered care in assisted living. *Journal of Aging & Social Policy, 10*(3): 7-26.

The Program of All-Inclusive Care for the Elderly (PACE): An Innovative Long-Term Care Model in the United States

Ada C. Mui, PhD, ACSW

Columbia University School of Social Work

SUMMARY. This article examines the long-term care service system in the United States, its problems, and an improved long-term care model. Problematic quality of care in institutional settings and fragmentation of service coordination in community-based settings are two major issues in the traditional long-term care system. The Program of All-Inclusive Care for the Elderly (PACE) has been emerging since the 1970s to address these issues, particularly because most frail elders prefer community-based to institutional care. The Balanced Budget Act of 1997 made

---

Dr. Ada Chan Yuk-Sim Mui is Associate Professor of Social Work at Columbia University School of Social Work, New York City. She received her Masters and PhD degrees in Social Work at Washington University in St. Louis. Her professional interests are social gerontology, family caregiving, long-term care, ethnicity and aging, elderly mental health and quality-of-life issues, and cross-cultural research methodology. Her publications include journal articles and book chapters that cover informal caregiving, formal service utilization, long-term care, and quality-of-life issues of frail older people. Her book, *Long-Term Care and Ethnicity*, published in 1998, examines the long-term care service delivery system and quality-of-life issues among frail older people in the United States.

Dr. Mui can be contacted at Columbia University School of Social Work, 622 West 113th St., New York, NY 10025, USA (E-mail: acm5@columbia.edu).

[Haworth co-indexing entry note]: "The Program of All-Inclusive Care for the Elderly (PACE): An Innovative Long-Term Care Model in the United States." Mui, Ada C. Co-published simultaneously in *Journal of Aging & Social Policy* (The Haworth Press, Inc.) Vol. 13, No. 2/3, 2001, pp. 53-67; and: *Long-Term Care in the 21st Century: Perspectives from Around the Asia-Pacific Rim* (ed: Iris Chi, Kalyani K. Mehta, and Anna L. Howe) The Haworth Press, Inc., 2001, pp. 53-67. Single or multiple copies of this article are available for a fee from The Haworth Document Delivery Service [1-800-HAWORTH, 9:00 a.m. - 5:00 p.m. (EST). E-mail address: getinfo@haworthpressinc.com].

PACE a permanent provider type under Medicare and granted states the option of paying a capitation rate for PACE services under Medicaid. The PACE model is a managed long-term care system that provides frail elders alternatives to nursing home life. The PACE program's primary goals are to maximize each frail elderly participant's autonomy and continued community residence, and to provide quality care at a lower cost than Medicare, Medicaid, and private-pay participants, who pay in the traditional fee-for-service system. In exchange for Medicare and Medicaid fixed monthly payments for each participating frail elder, PACE service systems provide a continuum of long-term care services, including hospital and nursing home care, and bear full financial risk. Integration of acute and long-term care services in the PACE model allows care of frail elders with multiple problems by a single service organization that can provide a full range of services. PACE's range of services and organizational features are discussed. *[Article copies available for a fee from The Haworth Document Delivery Service: 1-800-HAWORTH. E-mail address: <getinfo@haworthpressinc.com> Website: <http://www.HaworthPress.com> © 2001 by The Haworth Press, Inc. All rights reserved.]*

KEYWORDS. Capitation, community-based long-term care, long-term care, PACE

LONG-TERM CARE IN THE UNITED STATES

Many U. S. institutions, including those of education, employment, and health care, have felt the impact of the demographic trend of population aging for some time now. But with much larger numbers and increased life expectancy, long-term care for frail elders has emerged as one of the most important familial, social, and financial issues on the policy agenda. Further, because the family is the primary source of caregiving for frail elders, long-term care for elders has been and continues to be a serious issue for most American families. In this article, the author examines problems of the traditional long-term care system and introduces the Program of All-Inclusive Care for the Elderly (PACE)–a nationally recognized, innovative community-based long-term care model in the United States.

Demographic Trends

The need for long-term care in the United States is driven by interrelated trends in demography, prevalence of disability, and the role of informal caregivers vis-à-vis formal services. The United States experienced rapid demographic aging toward the end of the 20th century, with the population age 65 and older reaching 33.5 million, some 12.8% of the total population (Mui et al., 1998). This proportion is expected to remain near its current level over the next decade, but between 2010 and 2030, the baby boomers will join the older population. It is projected that by 2030, about 69.4 million Americans will be age 65 or older and that they will account for 20% of the population. Moreover, the most rapidly growing group is expected to be the 85+ population, with its current size doubling by 2025 and increasing fivefold by 2050, that is, from 3.6 million in 1995 to 18.2 million in 2050 (U. S. Bureau of the Census, 1996).

Longevity and Disability

While the majority of the community-dwelling population age 65 or older are disability-free, a strong positive association between advancing age and the prevalence of certain disabilities, as well as the link between some chronic diseases and subsequent disability, have been clearly demonstrated by Jette (1996). The proportion of people who have difficulties with any activity of daily living (ADL)–a common measure of functional limitations and disabilities in elders–increases rapidly with age, from only about 12% at ages 65-74 to 27% at ages 75-84 to 58% at age 85 or older.

Another indicator of the link between advancing age and disability is the rate of nursing home use in different age categories. In 1990, about 1% of persons between ages 65 and 74 were in nursing homes, with the percentage increasing to 6.1% of those between ages 75 and 84 and fully 24% of those age 85 or older (U. S. Bureau of the Census, 1993).

Although in general the morbidity rate among older persons has been decreasing (Manton, Stallard, & Corder, 1995), increasing life expectancy and the growth of the older population, especially those age 85 or older, will result in increasing numbers of disabled elders who need assistance in their daily lives. Recent projections are that the number of elderly needing long-term care will reach 10-14 million by 2020 and 14-24 million by 2060, compared with 7.3 million today (Manton, 1989; Mui et al., 1998; U. S. General Accounting Office [GAO], 1994). In 2018, it is estimated that 3.6 million elders will need nursing home beds, up 2 million from the current figure. Even more evident is the increasing number of families who will also face the daunting challenge of providing long-term care for their frail older relatives alongside other familial and job-related responsibilities.

What Is Long-Term Care?

To define long-term care, at least five components require clarification, namely, service types, funding sources, settings, service recipients, and service providers. Theoretically, long-term care services include a full continuum of care (e.g., acute medical services–inpatient and outpatient care, primary and specialty care, home health care; long-term care services–nursing home care, adult day care, respite, home care services; and social services–counseling, housing services, and many others). In terms of funding sources, formal services are usually paid for by public or private funding. Long-term care services can be provided through institutional (mostly nursing homes) or a wide variety of other community settings. The majority of frail elders who require long-term care services live in the community. Among the frail elderly population (7.3 million), only 1.6 million live in nursing homes, with 5.7 million receiving long-term care services in their homes or other community residential settings (U. S. General Accounting Office [GAO], 1996).

Who are the long-term care recipients? Long-term care services in the United States involve a wide range of health, personal care, and social services for people who need assistance in their daily lives because of chronic physical, functional, and/or mental disabilities and subsequent loss of the ability to function independently on a daily basis (Kane et al., 1998; Mui et al., 1998; U. S. GAO, 1996). All of these long-term care services may be provided by formal systems and/or unpaid informal caregivers. In both institutional and community settings, long-term care usually comes from a mix of unpaid informal sources, primarily family members, and formal sources supported by public and private funds. There has been a great deal of debate on the question of whether these two sources of care are compensatory, substituting for each other, or reciprocal; the answers that have been advanced are not yet clear. What is clear, and has not changed for decades, is that unpaid informal support from family and friends is the most prevalent form of long-term care. The informal system of support for frail elders is the backbone of long-term care, but these elders receive very few direct supportive services in the long-term care system (Kane et al., 1998). Currently, more than 90% of noninstitutionalized frail elders receive some informal care, while 67% depend exclusively on family and friends for care (National Academy on Aging, 1997). The engagement of formal services is prompted mainly by deterioration in the elder's level of independence, with a strong, direct correlation between the severity of disability and formal service utilization (Mui, Choi, & Monk, 1998).

Problems with the Long-Term Care Service System

Quality of care and fragmentation of service delivery are two major problems associated with the long-term care system in the United States. Historically, long-term care services are commonly compared in two broad categories, based on the setting in which formal services are delivered: institution-based services, delivered primarily to elders living in traditional nursing homes, and home- and community-based services, delivered to those living in the community. The most serious problem associated with services provided in a nursing home setting is poor quality of care. In the United States, long-term care can be very costly, especially in an institutional setting. In 1998, the average cost of nursing home care was about $56,000 but the quality of care has been documented to be problematic (U. S. GAO, 1996). While the state and federal governments have grappled with ways of improving the quality of care in nursing homes for more than two decades, effective quality-assurance mechanisms fall short of giving families comfort and confidence in the care their elderly relatives receive.

The bulk of public dollars spent in institutional care does not accomplish better quality-of-life outcomes for nursing home residents either (Mui et al., 1998). Research also indicates that most frail elders are unwilling to stay in a nursing home even if necessary. Data show that most frail elders in the community prefer death to entering a nursing home for long-term care (Mui & Burnette, 1994). Institutionalization restricts elders' sense of freedom, autonomy, flexibility, and sense of choice (Kane et al., 1998). The rigid routine of a nursing home has a significant negative impact on residents' morale. They may feel a sense of abandonment, powerlessness, and helplessness. Informal caregivers may feel a strong sense of failure or guilt. Quality of life of both the frail elder and his or her informal caregivers may worsen due to the elder's institutionalization.

Most frail elders prefer to stay at home to receive community-based long-term care services, but the major problem is a serious fragmentation of services coordination and a weak link in the continuum of care. Service organizations and service delivery systems often have gaps in the continuum of care (Branch, 2001). In most cases, the frail elder or the informal caregiver has to negotiate with the system and manage to get services to meet the frail elder's needs. Direct services and support to the informal caregivers are not sufficient. Most informal caregivers are heavily burdened emotionally because they not only provide the majority of the informal care but also play an important role in obtaining and managing services from paid sources (Binstock, Cluff, & von Mering, 1996). Research data point out that informal caregiving does not end when formal services begin (Mui & Burnette, 1994). Many families continue to provide supplemental caregiving for their relatives in nursing homes (Aneshensel, Pearlin, Mullan, Zarit, & Whitlatch, 1995; George & Maddox, 1989) and contribute to out-of-pocket payments, which accounted for nearly 36% of all long-term care expenditures in 1993 (U. S. GAO, 1996). Although many family members readily make themselves available to care for their dependent elderly relatives out of love and a sense of commitment, caregiving often creates physical, emotional, and financial strains on the younger generation when caregiving duties conflict with their family life and employment as well as draining their individual and family financial resources (Mui, 1992, 1993, 1995a, 1995b, 1995c; Mui & Morrow-Howell, 1993). Currently, about 2 million working Americans provide significant levels of unpaid care to elderly relatives who live in the community and need assistance with everyday activities.

NEED FOR AN IMPROVED COMMUNITY-BASED LONG-TERM CARE SYSTEM

With most frail elders preferring community to nursing home care, the demand for home- and community-based services is increasing, and this increase brings more attention to the improvement of program design, especially service integration. Many of the community-based long-term care programs implemented in the 1980s have been found to be cost-effective (Weissert et al., 1997). However, a considerable amount of research literature suggests that provision of noninstitutional services has generally raised health care costs because the limited reductions in institutional use are more than offset by the increased use of community-based long-term care (Hennessy & Hennessy, 1990; Wiener, 1990).

Use of home- and community-based long-term care relies in large part on the availability of both informal and formal caregivers. Much of the research focused on the relationship between informal and formal care has been driven by the concern, largely unsubstantiated, that increased access to formal care would replace the informal care given by family and friends who currently provide the majority of long-term care at no cost to government (Wiener, 1990).

Research on how better to integrate informal and formal care systems has been scarce, even though an informal support system is the backbone of long-term care for a frail elder (Kane et al., 1998). While informal caregivers are essential to understanding the needs and preferences of many elderly persons, some believe that health care professionals do not know how effectively to collaborate with an older person's informal support system. It is argued that neither Medicare nor Medicaid provides incentives for meaningful coordination of formal services and integration with informal care.

Many in the United States have challenged the long-term care system for years. To address the problematic issues related to the long-term care system, an improved long-term care service delivery model has been tested for more than a decade. The development of new service-delivery models that link both formal long-term care services and acute care, and that recognize the important role of informal care, has been the subject of some experimentation. One model that has achieved the desired outcome is the Program of All-Inclusive Care for the Elderly, now widely known as the PACE model. PACE is a managed long-term care system.

The primary goals of PACE are to maximize each frail elderly participant's autonomy and continued community residence and to provide quality care at a lower cost than Medicare, Medicaid, and private-pay participants, who pay in the traditional fee-for-service system. From the perspective of the federal government, the goal is to reduce the fragmentation of services and effectively integrate acute care and long-term care into a comprehensive, one-stop system (Hansen, 1999). In PACE, preventive and rehabilitative services are emphasized to stabilize and maintain chronic conditions and reduce complications of disease, thereby improving the quality of life of frail elders in the program and supporting their informal caregivers.

Growth of the PACE Model

The first PACE program, On Lok, was developed in 1971 in San Francisco's Chinatown by a community agency also called On Lok, Cantonese for "peaceful happy abode." The program was modeled after the British day hospital concept, with the service providers believing that frail elderly persons with multiple medical conditions could avoid institutionalization and continue to live in the community if home- and/or community-based medical and social services could be provided (Lee et al., 1998). The innovative PACE model "sets the pace" for alternatives to life in a nursing home (On Lok website, 2001). On Lok data also showed that the cost of care for frail elders in PACE was 15% less than in the traditional fee-for-service care system. In 1983, On Lok received waivers from Medicare and Medicaid to test its new financing method for long-term care: a form of risk-based capitation. In exchange for fixed monthly payments from Medicare and Medicaid for each participating frail elder, On Lok provided a continuum of services, including hospital and nursing home care, and bore full financial risk. In 1986, On Lok obtained a permanent Medicare and Medicaid waiver. Since then, On Lok has had no cost overruns and has been able to place up to 5% of its operating revenues in a risk reserve fund each year. The Balanced Budget Act of 1997 made PACE a permanent provider type under Medicare and granted states the option of paying a capitation rate for PACE services under Medicaid. The federal and state governments both achieve savings through the PACE program: Medicare saves about 5% and Medicaid saves up to 15% (On Lok Website, 2001). Currently, On Lok operates seven days a week, 52 weeks a year, serving more than 869 frail elders in the community throughout San Francisco. Evaluation data show that the PACE model of care provides a better quality of life to the frail elderly participants (Gelfand, 1999).

Legislation was passed to approve replication of the PACE model through federal demonstration sites in 1986. The first 10 sites began to provide community-based long-term care services in 1987. The number of PACE programs grew gradually in the 1990s until, by the end of 1998, there were 17 programs operating under dual Medicare and Medicaid capitation (payment of a fixed amount per client), with 14 pre-PACE programs in development (these sites receive Medicaid capitation for long-term care services and get fee-for-service reimbursement for Medicare services). In 2001, more than 70 organizations in 30 states are working in various stages of PACE development. Between 1990 and 1997, PACE and pre-PACE programs served almost 9,000 frail elders per year (Hansen, 1999; Irvin, Massey, & Dorsey, 1999).

Range of Services Provided in PACE

The one-stop comprehensive service package offered in PACE includes all Medicare and Medicaid services as well as community long-term care medical and social services, with no benefit limitations, co-payments, or deductibles. The integration of acute and long-term care services allows frail elders with multiple problems to be cared for by a single service organization that can provide a full range of needed services. PACE thus provides a "one-door" single point of entry to a comprehensive care package of preventive, acute, and long-term care services to allow frail elderly persons to live in the community as long as possible (Hooyman & Kiyak, 1999). PACE also provides specialized expertise in developing a care plan tailored to the individual's needs. The care plan takes into account the elderly person's medical condition, mental functioning, living environment, and the quality and quantity of the person's informal support system.

Informal and family support is the most important component to determine the success of the PACE model. For an elderly person too frail to live alone, a PACE program must rely on an informal support system to provide supervision and care during the hours when the frail elder is not at the adult day health center (ADHC). In PACE programs that provide housing services, the option of providing an elderly person with an apartment has created less reliance on informal support. PACE services, including primary care, social work, and restorative therapy, are provided in the PACE adult day health center, at home, in the hospital, and in the nursing home. PACE includes specialty and ancillary medical services as well as community-based long-term care services such as transportation, meals, home care, and personal care.

Distinguishing Organizational Features of PACE

While there are some variations among sites, the PACE approach has some shared distinguishing features (Hansen, 1999; Irvin, Massey, & Dorsey, 1999).

Client enrollment is restricted to nursing-home-eligible frail elders, age 55 and older, who choose to receive long-term care services in the community. Compared to other elderly populations, participants in PACE are similar to nursing home residents. The typical frail older population in PACE averages age 80 years or older, with about 30% of them age 85 or older. Typically, they have at least three ADL impairments and an average of 7.8 chronic medical conditions; almost 70% are mentally impaired, including those with dementia and depression. Nationally, PACE serves an ethnically diverse population, with 45% Caucasian, 26% African American, 15% Hispanic, 12% Asian/Pacific Islander, and 2% other, with the racial and ethnic distribution of each program reflecting the characteristics of the community served.

Funding. Under the Balanced Budget Act of 1997, PACE became a permanent provider through capitation payments from Medicare and Medicaid funds. Enrollment in PACE is limited to nursing-home-eligible frail elders who are dually entitled to Medicare and Medicaid programs or who have the financial resources to pay a premium equal to the Medicaid capitation rate.

The adult day health center (ADHC) is the central service-delivery site, especially for primary medical care services such as provision of a doctor or nurse specialist for assessment and/or treatment. The proportion of PACE participants utilizing primary medical care at the ADHC is around 90%, which is pretty high. All rehabilitation services are also provided in the ADHC. In the last quarter of 1992, most PACE program sites averaged between 1.4 and 3.5 days of rehabilitation per client, and between 52% and 88% of program participants utilized rehabilitation services in the ADHC.

Housing is a crucial component in the continuum of services at a majority of PACE sites, especially for those without family support. Most PACE programs have a waiting list for housing, ranging from four months to two years, and most programs have plans to develop housing services in the future.

Hospitalization can increase costs that are potentially damaging to the PACE program, so control of hospital utilization is very critical to the management of PACE risks. During a typical month, hospital use varies from 7% to 33% and nursing home use ranges from 1.2 to 2.2 days per client for most PACE programs.

Skilled home health services also have low utilization, approximately 2.4 hours per month per participant across PACE sites. Homemaker/personal care hours are much higher with an average of 10 to 17 hours per month per client.

A multidisciplinary team is the core professional group that provides case-management services. The program director serves as the facilitator of the intake and assessment meetings, and some sites have an executive director. Sometimes, the clinical managers (e.g., R.N.s, social workers) rotate the position of facilitator. In some cases, the program director also functions as executive director to facilitate the intake and assessment meetings. The multidisciplinary team typically includes ADHC supervisors, physicians, nurses, social workers, home health supervisors, physical therapists and/or occupational therapists and recreational therapists, home health nurses or aides, pharmacists, and other clinical specialists including psychologists and/or psychiatrists, dental clinicians, nursing home staff, durable medical equipment suppliers, hospice staff, and housing personnel. Some PACE programs have chaplains on staff to provide spiritual support to the participants, and they also attend the intake and assessment meetings. In terms of staffing intensity, a typical PACE program has one-third to one-half clinicians.

Evaluation Outcomes

PACE programs have been evaluated, and the results reported favorable outcomes in enrollment, cost saving, case-management quality, and effective multidisciplinary approach.

Cost outcomes. Data from the evaluation show that savings are possible. In 1998, the monthly Medicare capitation payment to PACE programs varied from $877 to $1,775 per participant, indicating that PACE services are more cost-effective than nursing home services. PACE funding arrangements are flexible enough to meet the needs of frail elders because all payments are pooled by the PACE sites to provide all needed services without traditional restrictions. PACE programs need to manage financial risk by keeping frail elders as healthy as possible through aggressive health prevention programs as well as careful supervision and monitoring in the clinic, center, and home. There are strong incentives to save money so that starting new programs or expanding existing services is possible. The prevalence of significant chronic medical conditions in the PACE population points to the importance of aggressive prevention strategies aimed at reducing hospitalization or nursing home placement (Hansen, 1999; Kane et al., 1998; Mui et al., 1998).

Best multidisciplinary team practice and service coordination. Upon admission to a PACE program, a frail older person is assessed systematically by the multidisciplinary team of clinicians responsible for service decisions. The team provides ongoing assessment, treatment planning, service provision, and monitoring. The focus of the frail older person's care plan is primary, secondary, and tertiary prevention. Careful coordination of needed services is achieved by team management of all PACE core services provided in the ADHC.

Enrollment. Most PACE programs serve 100 to 120 frail elderly participants and have a daily attendance of 60 to 70. The average number of clients in PACE sites that have operated four or more years is 375. The first and largest program, On Lok, had an enrollment of 793 participants as of December 1, 1998. Compared with other frail elders, those opting to enroll in PACE are more likely to be female, are more likely to have low incomes and less education, and are less likely to own homes. PACE frail elders require more assistance with IADLs but a similar level of assistance with ADLs. Most important, compared to non-PACE frail elders with a similar level of functional impairment and medical conditions, PACE participants use hospitals and nursing homes less, due mainly to PACE's early and timely comprehensive community care. PACE participants also have better health outcomes in terms of better health status and quality of life, and lower mortality rates.

LESSONS LEARNED, PROBLEMS REMAINING

Beyond the positive medical and quality-of-life outcomes associated with PACE programs, a number of broader lessons can be learned from the process of PACE development (Hansen, 1999; Kane et al., 1998; Mui et al., 1998). The first is that it takes time to change the system. Development of the PACE program took 25 years from the initial program idea to legislation and nationwide implementation.

Second, collaboration and cooperation among all planners and clinicians are keys to success. Since PACE's inception, one of its important features has been collaboration among program planners and providers, private funding agencies, foundations, and the government. In other words, multisector collaboration is critical and serves as a catalyst for system change. A new culture in collaboration had to be developed. President Harry S. Truman once said, "It is amazing what you can accomplish if you do not care who gets the credit," and that spirit seems to characterize the commitment and cooperation shown by those who have been involved in development of the PACE model.

Third, PACE has benefited from the cumulative collective wisdom of the multidisciplinary team. Beginning at the grassroots level, and using an "each one teach one" approach to replicate itself (Hansen, 1999), the PACE approach is a summary product of many past successes and failures experienced in the real world of operations. Examples of these benefits are the early evaluation of the On Lok model; technical assistance provided by On Lok to the replication sites; the design and creation of the PACE Minimum Data Set, which allowed sites to develop patient records in systematic ways and compare data among sites; integrative seminar and cross-site activities, including meetings, conferences, and other training; and development of standards of quality care, as the first steps toward accreditation of PACE service providers.

Fourth, the costs of system change have to be recognized, particularly the trade-off between short-term pain and long-term gain. The professional planners behind PACE recognized the importance of scientific data for program development, evaluation, and decision-making. Since the beginning of the PACE program, funding has been allocated to collect data and continue to develop a feasible, adequate information infrastructure. These resources included early "program-based, policy-oriented" research studies, cross-site data-collection protocols, reliability evaluation, computerized information systems, and regular evaluation reports with comparative information on program outcomes. PACE has grown up along with the information technology industry, and PACE, with assistance from the private and government sectors, has indeed kept pace.

The final and most important lesson of the PACE model development is the value of having the courage to change. PACE development and implementation required a complete reconfiguration of the traditional service-delivery system and a completely new way of caring for frail elders using an interdisciplinary professional team. Strong commitment to the team approach is necessary, as well as having a team all of whose members are competent and strong in their individual disciplines and have the skills and attitudes to work collaboratively to achieve broader objectives to enhance the favorable medical and psychosocial outcomes of the frail elders.

What problems, then, remain to be addressed if the PACE approach is to continue to advance? First, training of medical and allied health professionals is needed. PACE programs are growing in number and in size, and there is a pressing need for educational programs to ensure that appropriately trained professionals are available to care for the growing numbers of frail elders in the community.

Second, housing needs and services of the frail elderly population must be addressed. PACE programs are not responsible for housing in the sense of housing being a formal program benefit; payment for housing is not included in Medicare and Medicaid capitated reimbursements. In many cases, the lack of appropriate housing is the primary obstacle to an individual's survival in the community. PACE programs evaluate the frail elders' housing needs and help them secure housing services if possible.

Third and most fundamentally, care and support must be given to the informal caregivers of frail elders. Because PACE programs rely on voluntary participation of frail older people, they may encounter difficulties in recruiting potential participants with the most limitations in ADLs. Recruitment of frail elders may need to reach out to their family caregivers because informal caregivers usually serve as the link between the agency and the frail elders. Only through such collaboration with informal caregivers can PACE deliver formal services that are integrated with informal care.

PACE AND OTHER LONG-TERM CARE WEBSITES IN THE UNITED STATES

*National PACE Association (*http://www.natlpaceassn.org*):* Provides information on public policy, quality and research initiatives, and educational opportunities for those concerned with the well-being of frail elderly and the PACE model of care.
*On Lok Senior Health in San Francisco (*http://www.onlok.org*):* The first PACE program in the United States.
*Health Care Financing Administration (*http://www.hcfa.gov): Information on Medicare, Medicaid Programs in the United States.

REFERENCES

Aneshensel, C. S., Pearlin, L. I., Mullan, J. T., Zarit, S. H., & Whitlatch, C. J. (1995). *Profiles in caregiving: The unexpected career.* San Diego: Academic Press.
Binstock, R. H., Cluff, L. E., & von Mering, O. (1996). Issues affecting the future of long-term care. In R. H. Binstock, L. E. Cluff, & O. von Mering (Eds.), *The future of long-term care: Social and policy issues* (pp. 3-18). Baltimore: Johns Hopkins University Press.
Branch, L. G. (2001). Community long-term care services: What works and what doesn't? *The Gerontologist, 41*(3): 305-306.
Gelfand, D. E. (1999). *The aging network: Programs and services* (5th eds.). New York: Springer Publishing Company.
George, L. K., & Maddox, G. (1989). Social and behavioral aspects of institutional care. In M. Ory & K. Bond (Eds.), *Aging and health care: Social science and health perspectives* (pp. 116-141). London: Routledge.

Hansen, J. C. (1999). Practical lessons for delivering integrated services in a changing environment: The PACE model. *Generations*, *23*(2): 22-28.

Harrington, C., Carrillo, H., Mullen, J., & Swan, J. H. (1998). Nursing facility staffing in the States: The 1991 to 1995 period. *Medical Care Research and Review*, *55*(3), 334-363.

Hennessy, C. H., & Hennessy, M. (1990). Community-based long-term care for the elderly: Evaluation practice reconsidered. *Medical Care Review*, *47*(2): 221-259.

Hooyman, N. R., & Kiyak, H. A. (1999). *Social gerontology: A multidisciplinary perspective* (Fifth edition). Boston, MA: Allyn and Bacon.

Institute of Medicine (1986). *Committee on Nursing Home Regulation: Improving the quality of care in nursing homes.* Washington: National Academy Press.

Irvin, C. V., Massey, S., & Dorsey, T. (1999). Determinants of enrollment among applicants to PACE. *Health Care Financing Review*, *19*(2): 135-153.

Jette, A. M. (1996). Disability trends and transitions. In R. H. Binstock & L. K. George (Eds.), *Handbook of aging and the social sciences* (pp. 94-116). San Diego: Academic Press.

Kane, R. A., & Kane, R. L. (1987). *Long-term care: Principles, programs, and policies.* New York: Springer.

Kane, R. A., Kane, R. L., & Lodd, R. C. (1998). *The heart of long-term care.* New York: Oxford University Press.

Lee, W., Eng, C., Fox., N., & Etienne, M. (1998). PACE: A model for integrated care of frail older patients. *Geriatrics*, *53*(6): 62-74.

Manton, K. (1989). Epidemiological, demographic, and social correlates of disability among the elderly. *The Milbank Quarterly*, *67*, Supplement Part 1: 59-92.

Manton, K., Stallard, E., & Corder, L. (1995). Changes in morbidity and chronic disability in the U.S. elderly population: Evidence from the 1982, 1984, and 1989 National long-term care surveys. *Journal of Gerontology*, *50B*(4): S194-S204.

Mui, A. C. (1995a). Multidimensional predictors of caregiver strain among older persons caring for their frail spouses. *Journal of Marriage and the Family*, *57*: 733-740.

Mui, A. C. (1995b). Determinants of perceived health and functional limitations in elderly caregivers of frail spouses. *Journal of Aging and Health*, *7*(2): 283-300.

Mui, A. C. (1995c). Caring for frail elderly parents: A comparison of adult sons and daughters. *The Gerontologist*, *35*(1): 86-93.

Mui, A. C. (1993). The effects of caregiving on the emotional well-being of American older caregivers. *Hong Kong Journal of Gerontology*, *7*(1): 14-20.

Mui, A. C., & Burnette, D. (1994). Long-term care service use by frail elders: Is ethnicity a factor? *The Gerontologist*, *34*(2): 190-198.

Mui, A. C., & Morrow-Howell, N. (1993). Sources of emotional strain among the oldest old caregivers: Differential experiences of siblings and spouses. *Research on Aging*, *15*(1): 50-69.

Mui, A. C. (1992). Caregiver strain among black and white daughter caregivers: A role theory perspective. *The Gerontologist*, *32*(2), 203-212.

Mui A. C., Choi, N. G., & Monk, A. (1998). *Long-term care and ethnicity.* Westport, CT: Greenwood Press.

National Academy on Aging (1997). *Facts on long-term care.* Washington, DC.

On Lok Website (2001). http://www.onlok.org.

U.S. General Accounting Office (GAO). (1994). *Long term care: Diverse, growing population includes millions of Americans of all ages.* GAO/HEHS-95-26. Washington, DC: U.S. Government Printing Office.

U.S. General Accounting Office (GAO). (1996). *Long term care: Current issues and future directions.* GAO/HEHS-95-109. Washington, DC: The U.S. Government Printing Office.

U.S. Bureau of the Census. (1993). *Nursing home population, 1990.* CPH-L-137. Washington, DC: U.S. Government Printing Office.

U.S. Bureau of the Census. (1996). *Population projections of the United States by age, sex, race, and Hispanic origin: 1995 to 2050.* Current population reports, P24-1130. Washington, DC: U.S. Government Printing Office.

Weissert, W. G., Lesnick, T., Musliner, M., & Foley, K. A. (1997). Cost savings from home and community-based services: Arizona's capitated Medicaid long-term care program. *Journal of Health Politics, Policy and Law, 22*(6): 1329-1357.

Wiener, J. M. (1990). Myths and realities: Why most of what everybody knows about long-term care is wrong. Paper presented at the Executive Leadership Seminar, "Financing national health care: Tradeoffs between access and cost control." Washington, DC. The Brookings Institute, May 1990.

Williamson, J. L. (1999). The siren song of the elderly: Florida nursing homes and the dark side of chapter 400. *American Journal of Law and Medicine, 25*(2/3): 423-443.

Long-Term Care Funding in Canada: A Policy Mosaic

John P. Hirdes, PhD

University of Waterloo
Waterloo, ON, Canada

SUMMARY. When Canada was founded, health care was delegated as a provincial responsibility. Although the federal government shares a portion of health care costs, it is not directly responsible for the planning, delivery, and governance of health services. The 1984 Canada Health Act set national standards for the provision of physician and hospital services, but it does not apply to home care and long-term care facilities. Consequently, each province has established a unique approach to long-term care, resulting in a health policy mosaic. This paper examines different approaches to funding long-term care with a particular emphasis on the impacts of regionalization and of the implementation of case-mix-based funding systems. *[Article copies available for a fee from The Haworth Document Delivery Service: 1-800-HAWORTH. E-mail address: <getinfo@haworthpressinc.com> Website: <http://www.HaworthPress.com> © 2001 by The Haworth Press, Inc. All rights reserved.]*

John P. Hirdes is Associate Professor, Department of Health Studies and Gerontology at the University of Waterloo in Waterloo, Ontario, Canada. He is also Scientific Director at the Homewood Research Institute, Homewood Health Centre in Guelph, Ontario, Canada.

Dr. Hirdes can be contacted at the Department of Health Studies and Gerontology, University of Waterloo, Waterloo, ON, Canada, N2L 3G1 (E-mail: hirdes@uwaterloo.ca).

[Haworth co-indexing entry note]: "Long-Term Care Funding in Canada: A Policy Mosaic." Hirdes, John P. Co-published simultaneously in *Journal of Aging & Social Policy* (The Haworth Press, Inc.) Vol. 13, No. 2/3, 2001, pp. 69-81; and: *Long-Term Care in the 21st Century: Perspectives from Around the Asia-Pacific Rim* (ed: Iris Chi, Kalyani K. Mehta, and Anna L. Howe) The Haworth Press, Inc., 2001, pp. 69-81. Single or multiple copies of this article are available for a fee from The Haworth Document Delivery Service [1-800-HAWORTH, 9:00 a.m. - 5:00 p.m. (EST). E-mail address: getinfo@haworthpressinc.com].

KEYWORDS. Long-term care, universal coverage, case-mix classification system, for-profit home care, not-for-profit home care

HISTORICAL CONTEXT FOR CANADIAN HEALTH POLICY

The characteristics of Canada's health care system for the elderly have their roots in the British North America Act, under which Canada was founded in 1867. Health care was assigned as a provincial responsibility at a time when expenditures in that area were negligible. At the turn of the 20th century, governments focused primarily on the establishment and administration of poor houses sheltering various populations including the frail elderly (Forbes et al., 1987). Private practitioners provided medical care to patients paying for their own expenses, but pressure for government to take a greater role in health care grew with the depression of the 1930s.

Publicly funded health care was introduced to Canada in 1957 through the federal government's Hospital Insurance and Diagnostic Services Act, followed by the Medical Care Act in 1966, which provided universal coverage for physician services. Health care was a responsibility shared by federal and provincial governments with both initially contributing equal funding. The primary role of the federal government has been to set national standards and provide funding through tax transfers to the provinces. The federal government provides direct health care services only to a small population of Canadians composed mainly of First Nations, members of the military, veterans, and the Royal Canadian Mounted Police. The delivery of health care is a provincial responsibility, but most provinces have further divested management of health services to the regional level.

The 1984 Canada Health Act was a policy landmark because it set uniform standards for hospital and medical services across the country. According to this legislation, each province is required to provide health services with the following characteristics:

- Access to medically necessary services without financial barriers;
- Portability of benefits from one province to another;
- Public administration of health insurance with provincial governments as the sole insurers for medically necessary services;
- Comprehensive coverage of all medically necessary services provided by hospitals, physicians, and dentists;
- Universality of coverage for all residents of Canada.

This legislation ensured that all Canadians had access to medical and hospital services when needed and that their benefits were transportable if they were to move from one region of the country to another. It also prevented the use of user fees or any other potential financial barriers to access to necessary services.

Canadians have come to view the health care system as a central component of their national identity distinguishing Canada from the United States. The principles of universal access have been an important source of pride for Canadians, but increasing fiscal constraints and service reductions have led to a rising concern about the long-term viability of the Canadian model of health care. There is growing anxiety over the implications of population aging with respect to its demands on health services, even though the evidence indicates that population aging has played at most a minor role in increases in health expenditures over the last two decades (Angus et al., 1995).

It is fair to say that the initial conceptualization of publicly funded health care up to and including the Canada Health Act was not based on a model that planned explicitly for the needs of an aging population. Despite universal coverage for hospital services and physician services, there is no federal legislation, nor are there national standards, for home care, long-term care facilities, or pharmaceutical benefits. These services are not covered by federal Medicare legislation and are instead delivered through a diverse mosaic of policies created on a province-by-province basis. Indeed, recent attempts by the federal government to introduce national home care and national pharmacare programs were dismissed by at least some provincial premiers as a federal government attempt to impose "boutique programs" on the provinces.

This federal policy gap has meant that Canadians experience substantial variability in funding models for long-term care from province to province (Béland & Shapiro, 1994; Greb et al., 1994; Hirdes & Berg, 1999). Some provinces allow for privately operated nursing homes, whereas others require only publicly operated, or charitable homes. Some provinces require a co-payment by residents of long-term care facilities, whereas others do not. The size of these co-payments also varies, with some provinces requiring residents to pay until assets are spent down. Other provinces require a co-payment that is geared to minimum income levels, for example, based on the Canada Pension Plan.

HEALTH EXPENDITURES IN CANADA

Health expenditures in Canada have been rising in absolute, per capita, and percentage of GDP terms (Canadian Institute for Health Information, 2001). The national health care budget currently stands at approximately $95 billion, or about $3000 Canadian (about $1,900 US) per individual. This represents

9.3% of Gross Domestic Product, placing Canada at among the more expensive publicly funded health care systems, but remaining well below U. S. expenditures on GDP health care.

The large majority of health expenditures are accounted for by hospital and physician services, and about 70% of these expenditures are from public sources. The bulk of private expenditures involves insurance coverage (often through employers) for dental, pharmaceutical, rehabilitation, and a limited range of alternative health services (e.g., chiropractic, massage therapy). Long-term care and other facilities represent less than 10% of national expenditures on health care. The introduction of Medicare meant that health expenditures in Canada stabilized in the late 1960s and 1970s, compared with ongoing escalations in costs in the United States. In the mid 1980s, a substantial jump in health expenditures occurred mainly as a function of wage inflation among health professionals, rising drug costs, and increased intensity of medical interventions (Angus et al., 1995; Barer et al., 1995). However, in response to rapidly growing deficits, the federal government imposed reductions in transfer payments to the provinces in the early 1990s, resulting in a leveling out of health expenditures. At the same time, a recession forced most provinces to impose reductions in health expenditures beyond the levels of reductions in federal transfer payments.

FUNDING FOR LONG-TERM CARE FACILITIES

It is impossible to describe in detail a *singular* long-term care policy framework that applies uniformly to each province and territory in the country (Havens, 1995). At the risk of oversimplification, it is probably more useful to focus on two main forces shaping long-term care funding policy in Canada: they are, first, regionalization and, second, the introduction of case-mix classification systems. On the latter issue, the present discussion will draw particularly on Ontario's approach to long-term care funding, but it must be recognized that no one province's experience can be fully generalized to the remaining provinces.

The Impact of Regionalization

Beginning in the early 1990s, most Canadian provinces introduced a new layer of government at the regional level that would be responsible for the planning and operation of health services within their jurisdictions (Canadian Institute for Health Information, 2001). Provincial governments transferred funding to local authorities to distribute among health care agencies and service providers in their districts. In contrast, Ontario chose not to implement regionalization and its Ministry of Health and Long-Term Care sets the operating budgets for hospitals, nursing homes, and homes for the aged on a facility-by-facility basis. (Nursing homes are generally private organizations providing long-term care on a for-profit basis, whereas homes for the aged are not-for-profit organizations run by charities or municipalities.)

The use of a population-based funding approach is most evident in provinces that have moved towards regional health authorities. Under this model, per capita allocation of funding may be adjusted by population characteristics in order to reflect the health care funding needs of a given region. In most cases, these formulae are reasonably simplistic, relying only on a limited set of attributes (e.g., age distributions) to set funding levels, but these are typically not tied to the current users of the health care system. That is, a region may be allocated a funding envelope based on the overall population aged 75+ years, but not the characteristics of persons actually using acute care, home care, long-term care, rehabilitation, or mental health services. Some provinces like Alberta have attempted to establish somewhat more complex descriptive systems to use with population-based funding approaches, but these are generally not applied at the provider/agency level.

The key problem with population-based funding is that it does not link explicitly the characteristics of users of health services with funding levels assigned to those organizations. If a regional government fails to differentiate among facilities or agencies that provide services to clientele with heavier and more complex care needs than peer organizations, there will continue to be a financial incentive at the provider level to differentially admit persons with light care needs. A second major problem is that age is, at best, a crude indicator of the need for health services, and it is of little use in differentiating persons who reside in the community instead of institutional settings. There are few indicators beyond age available on a consistent basis across jurisdictions to allow for more sophisticated funding models. For this reason, even in provinces that have implemented regionalized approaches to health care, there has been a growing interest in case-mix-based funding systems.

Case-Mix-Based Payment Systems for Long-Term Care

Global budgets characterized by flat rates based on historical funding levels are still evident in sectors like home care and psychiatry in most Canadian provinces. However, funding for long-term facilities is beginning to be based on case-mix data describing the relative resource intensity of facility residents. Although a number of provinces have developed rudimentary classification schemes based on residents' expected hours of nursing services needed, these are not always linked to facility level budgets. However, two case-mix systems used to calculate facility level costs in Canada are the Alberta Resident Classification System (ARCS) (Alberta Health, 1988) and the Resource Utilization Groups (RUG-III) (Fries et al., 1994).

The ARCS system was developed by Alberta Health as a means of describing the resource intensity of nursing home residents through a classification approach relying on abstracts from residents' charts done by external "assessors." Residents are classified into seven levels of care ranging from categories A through G, with higher-level categories being assigned higher levels of funding. The primary characteristics used to differentiate clients along this continuum are: bowel and urinary continence, four measures of activities of daily living, and two measures of behavior disturbance. The data sources for these assessments are the notes taken by nurses over the course of a year, which are evaluated once annually by individuals outside the organization who are not involved in the care of the resident. The ARCS scores assigned to each resident are not made available to administrators and are reported only in summary form to describe the case-mix score for the entire facility. Facility level results are often not reported until several months after the classification visit. This poses a significant challenge to nursing home administrators, who are sometimes informed of the need to make substantial budget cuts with only a few months notice prior to the onset of the new fiscal year. The reliance on resident charts as a primary information source and the absence of direct assessments by classifiers have made the ARCS system particularly vulnerable to gaming. The phrase "charting for dollars" has been coined in Ontario to describe the change in charting practices used by nurses in long-term care facilities to highlight characteristics of the ARCS system most likely to be associated with higher funding levels. The ARCS assessments are not used for any other applications, such as benchmarking exercises to evaluate the quality of care and outcomes.

Ontario and Saskatchewan have been the first two Canadian provinces to mandate the implementation of the Minimum Data Set 2.0 (MDS 2.0) assessment system for complex continuing care hospitals/units and nursing homes, respectively (Morris et al., 1995; Hirdes et al., 1999). The primary purpose for Ontario's implementation has been to use MDS as a data source for classifying complex continuing care hospitals/unit patients, according to the RUG-III system. The Department of Health in Saskatchewan also mandated the submission of MDS data in the form of RUG-III scores, but it is not yet clear whether those data will be used to set funding for health regions in that province. A more likely possibility is that the Department of Health will use this for general descriptive purposes, and the regions themselves may use the algorithm to allocate funding to their respective nursing homes.

The Ontario Ministry of Health completed a role study to evaluate the need for chronic hospitals/units in 1995 (Chronic Care Implementation Task Force, 1995). The province subsequently assigned the Ontario Joint Policy and Planning Committee (JPPC) the task of developing a recommendation for the assessment and classification system to be used for complex continuing care; "chronic hospital/unit" came to be referred to as "complex continuing care hospitals/units." The review focused on ARCS, RUG-III, and the Functional Independence Measure Function Related Groups (FIM-FRGs) (Stineman et al., 1994). However, given the absence of a published weighting system for FIM-FRGs at the time, the attention soon narrowed to ARCS and RUG-III. RUG-III was ultimately chosen as the funding system for complex continuing care because it was perceived to be more sensitive to clinical complexity, it had higher explained variance with respect to resource utilization, and there was better scientific evidence for its reliability and validity (see Hirdes et al., 1996; Hirdes, 1997 for more detailed discussion).

Ontario began using RUG-III as a basis for reimbursement to complex continuing care of hospitals/units in Spring 2001. It was initially used to specify allocations of an incentive bonus based on the relative efficiency in using hospital resources. That approach is now embedded in the hospital funding formula for complex continuing care. Unlike the ARCS system, RUG-III has the advantage that the data are gathered by the facility's own staff who are familiar with the needs of patients they are describing, and administrators have access to real time case-mix data at the individual patient level. Moreover, the widespread use of MDS data for measuring the quality of care based on indicators developed by Zimmerman et al. (1995) has the benefit that it counterbalances the tendency to game the case-mix system by over-stating certain clinical characteristics (e.g., pressure ulcers).

More recently, the governments of Nova Scotia, Manitoba, British Columbia, and the Yukon have undertaken similar evaluations of assessment systems for long-term care and come to the same conclusion as Ontario and Saskatchewan. However, in those provinces, the primary attraction to the MDS assessments system appears to be its applications for care planning and quality management, rather than funding alone.

KEY CHALLENGES IN FUNDING LONG-TERM CARE

National Inequalities in Long-Term Care Services

From a national perspective, among the most important problems facing Canadian long-term care are the regional disparities in the types of services available to Canadian seniors and unequal access to therapeutic interventions in home- or facility-based care. The different approaches in funding have had a direct impact on the types of services seniors receive, irrespective of their needs. For example, in a report prepared for the Ontario Ministry of Health and Long-Term Care, the Ontario Association of Non-Profit Homes and Services for Seniors, and the Ontario Long-Term Care Association (Hirdes et al., 2001), regional and cross-sectoral variations in funding were clearly associated with differential access to rehabilitation, mental health, and nursing services for Canadian nursing home residents. For example, residents of Ontario nursing homes were approximately seven times less likely to receive rehabilitation when they demonstrated the potential for improved functional ability compared to similar individuals in Ontario complex continuing care hospitals/units. Moreover, Ontario nursing home residents were often less likely to get these kinds of services than nursing home residents not only in Saskatchewan and Manitoba, but, as an international comparative study shows, also in Michigan, Mississippi, Maine, South Dakota, The Netherlands, Finland, and Sweden.

These regional disparities in funding systems also have a differential impact on the families of nursing home residents. For example, in Nova Scotia the resident is expected to spend down assets in order to pay for long-term care services. In Ontario, the same type of individual would only be expected to use personal income to pay for a co-payment representing less than one third of the cost of long-term care services.

The lack of a national standard for assessing residents of long-term care facilities has also made it difficult to make direct comparisons of the relative resource intensity of persons receiving institutionally-based long-term care services across Canada. In many cases, the complete absence of data makes it virtually impossible to compare the relative needs of long-term care facility residents in one province with those of another. As a result, differences in acuity levels generally are undetected, and one cannot be certain that there is a consistent pattern of service delivery in long-term care across Canada.

Managing Care in Diverse Settings

The use of different classification systems across sectors in Ontario has increased the complexity of funding long-term care services. As a result, the Ontario Health Services Restructuring Commission (HSRC) recommended in 1998 that the province adopt a single assessment and classification system for long-term care facilities and for complex continuing care based on the MDS. The adoption of this recommendation could be expected to reduce the above-mentioned cross-sectoral inequalities in access to health services.

An increased diversity of care settings also means that elderly individuals in Canada receive services from a large variety of service providers. Medicare was founded in a health care system that was comprised mainly of physicians and hospitals. However, in today's health care system, Ontario seniors with mental health problems may receive services from: community mental health organizations; for-profit or not-for-profit home care providers, contracted by single-point entry agencies known as Community Care Access Centres (CCACs); geriatric outreach teams based in hospitals; nursing homes; homes for the aged; retirement homes; complex continuing care hospitals/units; or geriatric psychiatry units/programs based in mental health facilities. This diversity in care providers may have the advantage that the system has more flexibility in responding to the needs of different kinds of individuals. On the other hand, it has also led to fragmentation of care delivery and inequality in access to services, because these different providers do not necessarily receive consistent levels of funding to provide services to individuals with similar types of needs.

Some provinces (e.g., Alberta) have considered the possibility of establishing a single cross-sectoral classification system that would aim to describe the resource intensity of individuals regardless of the sector of health care from which they receive services. While there is some intuitive appeal in the notion of person-specific measures of resource intensity, there are a number of important conceptual and practical limitations that would suggest a unitary case-mix classification system may be neither feasible nor appropriate for the entire health care system. For example, research by Hollander (2001) has shown that the relative resource weights of persons in long-term care facilities and in home care programs classified into the same groups by British Columbia's classification system are not the same. That is, the community- and institution-based individuals classified into the same level of care by the British Columbia system do not have the same relative order of magnitude of difference when compared with the same reference group. In addition, Bjorkgren et al. (2000) showed that Instrumental Activities of Daily Living (IADLs) are more important determinants of resource utilization in home care settings than Activities of Daily Living (ADLs). In contrast, Fries et al. (1994) showed that ADLs are among the most important determinants of resource utilization in nursing home settings. Similarly, research by Yamauchi et al. (1997) on case-mix systems for psychiatry has shown that mental health service utilization is determined primarily by patient characteristics like psychotic symptoms, suicidal tendencies, violence, and aggressive behavior. Therefore, the use of a cross-sectoral case-mix classification system would be unwieldy, because of its level of complexity and its need to use measures that are relevant to some, but not all, sectors.

Disentangling Case-Mix, Payment, and Eligibility Systems

Even if Ontario does implement the RUG-III system for both complex continuing care hospitals/units and long-term care facilities, additional work remains to establish a unified funding formula. One needs to differentiate between case-mix systems that classify individuals into different groups based on relative resource intensity, and payment systems that translate case-mix and other data into the funding envelope allocated to a specific organization. The formula for a payment system includes, but is not limited to, case-mix data (Ladak, 1998; Teare, 2000). Other factors to be considered include labor contracts that may specify different wage ranges, funding for drug costs, and special facility adjustments for locations in remote rural settings, or for teaching status.

It is also important to differentiate case-mix systems from eligibility systems (Béland & Shapiro, 1994). Although there will naturally be some overlap between case-mix measures and decisions related to eligibility for services, it should be clear that these represent different applications of long-term care data. Case-mix systems tend to deal with the relative costs of caring for specific types of individuals, whereas eligibility systems relate to the specific set of services and location of care that would be most appropriate for an individual. Economies of scale may dictate that certain rare, expensive groups of patients should be clustered together, making them eligible for a more resource-intensive kind of service. However, it may also be appropriate to care for individuals with the same level of resource intensity in different settings. For example, persons requiring palliative care may be relatively more resource-intensive than other clients in community settings, but their position in a case-mix distribution need not translate to placement in a specific institution. Factors other than cost alone should influence the choice of the location of care and types of services these individuals receive.

One of the more important recommendations made by the Ontario Health Services Restructuring Commission (HSRC) was an attempt to differentiate more clearly who should be placed in complex continuing care versus long-term care facilities. The guidelines set forth by the HSRC have resulted in admission patterns that have moved complex continuing care toward a greater emphasis on post-acute services with much shorter episodes of care (Teare et al., 2000). One consequence of this change is that the relative resource intensity of long-term care facility residents has also gone up, because these persons are no longer eligible for complex continuing care services. However, the Alberta Resident Classification System is not particularly well adapted to addressing the needs of this more clinically complex population. Even though there is a widely held view among long-term care facility administrators and policymakers that the resource intensity of nursing home and home for the aged residents has been going up, this is not reflected in provincial patterns for the ARCS system (Ontario Ministry of Health and Long-Term Care, 2000). For example, there has been a steady decline in the proportion of persons classified in the highest ARCS level of funding (category G) over the last five years. Therefore, there is a clear danger that the disparities between complex continuing care and long-term care in funding may be even further magnified, as persons who previously received complex continuing care services are located increasingly in long-term care facilities.

Systemic Consequences of Long-Term Care Funding

The issue of adequate funding for long-term care in facilities and in the community has the potential to have unintended negative consequences for the system as a whole. For example, if long-term care facilities receive inadequate funding to address the clinical complexities of persons seeking admission to long-term care, it may be more difficult to place them in the less expensive long-term care facilities compared with the acute care hospital beds they currently occupy. Similarly, length of stay in acute hospitals is likely to increase if home care programs do not have necessary resources to provide intensive services in the community. If facilities or community agencies are compelled to accept clients and residents for whom they have inadequate funding, one can expect the outcome and the quality of that care not to be of an appropriate standard. This may in fact lead to an exacerbation of care needs leading to higher costs over the long term.

CONCLUSION

Canada's universal, publicly funded health care system has not been designed in a way that established a uniform national approach to long-term care. Instead, the needs of the frail elderly are addressed through a policy mosaic that results in inequalities in access to services and differential burdens of care on family members. Moreover, the lack of a standardized health information system has made it difficult to compare the experiences of users of long-term care systems from province to province. The implementation of case-mix classification systems like RUG-III has the potential to improve funding approaches to long-term care, but much work remains before the needs of the frail elderly are addressed adequately and equitably across Canada.

REFERENCES

Alberta Health (1988). *Alberta Resident Classification System for long-term care facilities: Instructions for completing the Resident Classification Form.* Edmonton: Alberta.

Angus, D. E., Auer, L., Cloutier, J. E., & Albert, T. (1995). *Sustainable health care for Canada.* Ottawa: University of Ottawa.

Barer, M. L., Evans, R. G., & Hertzman, C. (1995). Avalanche or glacier? Health care and the demographic rhetoric. *Canadian Journal on Aging, 14*(2): 193-224.

Béland, F., & Shapiro, E. (1994). Ten provinces in search of a long-term care policy. In Marshall, V. W. & McPherson, B. D. (Eds.). *Aging: Canadian perspectives.* Toronto: Broadview Press.

Bjorkgren, M. A., Fries, B. E., & Shugarman, L. R. (2000). A RUG-III based case-mix system for home care. *Canadian Journal on Aging, 19*(suppl. 2): 106-125.

Canadian Institute for Health Information (2001). *Health care in Canada.* Ottawa: Canadian Institute for Health Information.

Chronic Care Implementation Task Force (1995). *Report of the Chronic Care Implementation Task Force.* Hamilton: Educational Centre for Aging and Health.

Forbes, W. F., Jackson, J. A., & Kraus, A. S. (1987). *Institutionalization of the elderly in Canada.* Toronto: Butterworths.

Fries, B. E., Schneider, D. P., Foley, J. W., Gavazzi, M., Burke, R., & Cornelius, E. (1994). Refining a case-mix measure for nursing homes: Resource Utilization Groups (RUG-III). *Medical Care, 32*: 668-685.

Greb, J., Chambers, L. W., Gafni, A., Goeree, R., & Labelle, R. (1994). Inter-provincial comparisons of public and private sector long-term care facilities for the elderly in Canada. *Canadian Public Policy, XX*(3): 278-296.

Havens, B. (1995). Long-term care diversity within the care continuum. *Canadian Journal on Aging, 14*(2): 245-262.

Health Services Restructuring Commission (HSRC) (1998). *Change and transition– Planning guidelines and implementation strategies for home care, long-term care, mental health, rehabilitation, and sub-acute care.* Toronto: Health Services Restructuring Commission.

Hirdes, J. P. (1997). Development of a cross-walk from the Minimum Data Set 2.0 to the Alberta Classification System. *Health Care Management Forum, 10*(1): 27-34.

Hirdes, J. P., & Berg, K. (1999). Canada. In Carpenter, G. I., Challis, D., Hirdes, J. P., Ljunggren, G., & Bernabei, R. (Eds.). *Care of older people: A comparison of systems in North America, Europe and Japan.* London: Farrand Press.

Hirdes, J. P., Botz, C. A., Kozak, J., & Lepp, V. (1996). Identifying an appropriate case-mix measure for chronic care: Evidence from an Ontario pilot study. *Healthcare Management Forum, 9*: 40-46.

Hirdes, J. P., Fries, B. E., Morris, J. N., Steel, K., Mor, V., Frijters, D., Jonsson, P., LaBine, S., Schalm, C., Stones, M. J., Teare, G., Smith, T., Marhaba, M., & Perez, E. (1999). Integrated health information systems based on the RAI/MDS series of assessment instruments. *Healthcare Management Forum, 12*(4): 30-40.

Hirdes, J. P., Fries, B. E., Frijters, D., & Teare, G. F. (2001). *Canadian, US and international comparisons of resource intensity and responses to the needs of residents in long-term care facilities.* Toronto: Technical report to the Ontario Long-Term Care Association, Ontario Ministry of Health and Ontario Association of Not-for-profit Homes and Services for Seniors.

Hirdes, J. P., Fries, B. E., Frijters, D., & Teare, G. (2001). Canadian, U.S., and international comparisons of resource intensity and responses to the needs of residents in long-term care facilities. Technical report to the Ontario Ministry of Health.

Hollander, M. (2001). Substudy 1: Comparative cost analysis of home care and residential care services. Victoria, BC: Centre on Aging, University of Victoria.

Ladak, N. (1998). *Understanding how Ontario hospitals are funded: An introduction.* Toronto: Joint Policy and Planning Committee.

Morris J. N., Hawes, C., Murphy, K., & Nonemaker, S. (1995). *Long-term care resident assessment instrument user's manual–Version 2.0.* Baltimore: Health Care Financing Administration.

Ontario Ministry of Health and Long-Term Care (2000). *Report of the long-term care facilities classification review.* Toronto: Ministry of Health and Long-Term Care.

Stineman M. G., Escarce, J. J., Goin, J. E., Hamilton, B. B., Granger, C. V., & Williams, S. V. (1994). A case mix classification system for medical rehabilitation. *Medical Care, 32*(4): 366-379.

Teare, G. F. (1999). *Cost per case-mix weighted activity for complex continuing care in Ontario–technical paper from the JPPC Complex Continuing Care Funding Working Group.* Toronto: JPPC, JPPC Reference Document RD #8-12.

Yamauchi, K. (1997). Designing a new payment system for psychiatric care: Developing a case-mix classification system. *Journal of the Japanese Society of Hospital Administration, 34*(2): 155-167.

Zimmerman D., Karon, S. L., Arling, G., Clark, B. R., Collins, T., Ross, R. et al. (1995). Development and testing of nursing home quality indicators. *Health Care Financing Review, 16*(4): 107-127.

National Consistency
and Provincial Diversity in Delivery
of Long-Term Care in Canada

Peter Chan, MSW, MPH

Program Manager, Richmond Health Services Society
British Columbia, Canada

S. R. Kenny, BSc, MHSA

Executive Director,
British Columbia Health Industry Development Office

Peter Chan is Program Manager, Diagnostic Services, at The Richmond Hospital, Canada. He is an experienced practitioner in aged care services. He received his Master of Social Work and Master of Public Health from the University of Hawaii at Manoa in 1980. He has been involved in many consultancy projects commissioned by the Hong Kong Government and social service agencies since 1993.

Mr. Chan can be contacted at Health and Welfare Bureau, Hong Kong Government, Garden Road, Central Hong Kong (E-mail: peterhtchan@hotmail.com).

Steve Kenny has been Executive Director of the British Columbia Health Industry Development Office for the last five years. The Office is a public-sector, non-profit agency that is responsible for managing international health projects with expertise from British Columbia's public and private health sectors. Prior to this current role, Mr. Kenny held several senior positions with the British Columbia Ministry of Health from 1982-94. These include Executive Director of the Medical Services Plan, which is responsible for reimbursement of physicians for all medical services provided to BC residents, and Executive Director of Hospital Care, which provides funding, standards, and monitoring for all hospitals in the Province. He was also Assistant Deputy Minister responsible for hospital care, long-term care, services to the elderly, ambulance services, and facilities planning and construction.

Mr. Kenny has his Masters of Health Services Administration from the University of Alberta. Mr. Kenny can be contacted at BCHIDO/CAMSI, 2170 Mt. Newton X Rd., Saanichton, British Columbia, Canada V8M 2B2 (E-mail: skenny@caphealth.org).

[Haworth co-indexing entry note]: "National Consistency and Provincial Diversity in Delivery of Long-Term Care in Canada." Chan, Peter, and S. R. Kenny. Co-published simultaneously in *Journal of Aging & Social Policy* (The Haworth Press, Inc.) Vol. 13, No. 2/3, 2001, pp. 83-99; and: *Long-Term Care in the 21st Century: Perspectives from Around the Asia-Pacific Rim* (ed: Iris Chi, Kalyani K. Mehta, and Anna L. Howe) The Haworth Press, Inc., 2001, pp. 83-99. Single or multiple copies of this article are available for a fee from The Haworth Document Delivery Service [1-800-HAWORTH, 9:00 a.m. - 5:00 p.m. (EST). E-mail address: getinfo@haworthpressinc.com].

83

SUMMARY. The aim of this article is to demonstrate the diversity in delivery of long-term care at the provincial level, within a national legislative framework that provides universal health insurance and public administration. Not all provinces have legislated provision of long-term care, but mandates for provincial long-term care programs typically address the needs of those with chronic health needs and maintain them in the community for as long as possible. Eligibility is based on common criteria of residency, health need, facility, assessment, and consent. The three common components of the service delivery system are institutional care, community-based services, and home-based services; the kinds of services within each component and the mix among them vary from province to province. There are also five common features in provincial service delivery systems: single point of entry, assessment, client classification, case management, and single administration. Throughout the article, examples from different provinces show the varying ways in which these aspects of service delivery have been addressed, and recent innovations have furthered this diversity. A detailed account of quality management systems also shows that while all provinces have adopted a common set of principles, they use a range of methods to pursue quality of care and to promote good practice. *[Article copies available for a fee from The Haworth Document Delivery Service: 1-800-HAWORTH. E-mail address: <getinfo@haworthpressinc.com> Website: <http://www.HaworthPress.com> © 2001 by The Haworth Press, Inc. All rights reserved.]*

KEYWORDS. Assessment, client classification, innovation, not-for-profit providers, quality of care

ROLES OF CENTRAL AND PROVINCIAL GOVERNMENTS

Canada has a long-established framework of national, public provision of health and social services and a tradition of joint responsibility shared between the federal and provincial governments. This framework provides for a degree of national consistency at the same time as allowing diversity of outcomes at the provincial level, and the aim of this article is to demonstrate the interplay of central and provincial influences on the delivery of long-term care.

Federal legislation was introduced to provide hospital coverage for the population in 1957, and in 1968, medical care legislation provided for the coverage of medically necessary physician care. In both cases, these Acts provided that the federal government would share in the costs of health care delivered by the provinces on a 50% basis. In 1977, the Established Programs Financing Act changed the cost-sharing arrangement so that the provinces were block funded, primarily on a population basis rather than on a percentage of overall expenditures. These programs cover the aged along with all other age groups.

In 1984, the Canada Health Act reinforced the five principles of health insurance, namely: universality, providing coverage for all eligible residents; comprehensiveness, ensuring a full range of hospital and medical services; accessibility, removing barriers to access to care, including point-of-service costs; portability, requiring each province to cooperate and provide care to residents of any other province; and public administration by a non-profit, public sector body.

Against the background of a uniform national legislative framework, two factors contribute to diversity in outcomes for provincial long-term care systems. First, since the Established Programs Financing Act, the provinces have had the incentive, but not necessarily the requirement, to provide additional health services other than hospital and medical. Such programs were introduced mainly to reduce the cost of the more expensive medical and hospital services and thus the overall cost of health care. As part of their responses, five of the ten provinces have passed legislation to introduce long-term care programs; for example, British Columbia's Continuing Care Act passed in 1978 enabled a full-service, long-term care program. In provinces that do not have similar legislation, long-term care services and programs are delivered under the authority of government policy.

A second source of diversity in long-term care systems is the differing sizes and compositions of the provincial populations and their social and economic circumstances, as documented by the National Advisory Council on Aging (1999). Of Canada's total population of some 30 million, over 10 million live in Ontario, while Prince Edward Island has a total population of only 130,000. A major contrast for service delivery is between the highly urbanized provinces and those with low population densities and dispersed rural settlements. While this article gives an overview of diversity, many detailed studies of long-term care programs in individual provinces are available; the development of programs in British Columbia, the third largest province with four million people, can be traced through reports from the provincial Ministry of Health and Ministry Responsible for Seniors (1992), as well as more recent evaluations (Hollander & Pallan, 1995).

Provincial Responsibilities for Long-Term Care Programs

In each province, the overall responsibility for long-term care programs rests with the Ministry of Health. In several provinces, the Ministry responsible for health may also have the responsibility for other services such as social or community services. The provinces normally retain the right to determine funding issues, quality and standards, services to be provided, and eligibility of clients to receive long-term care services. The mandate of long-term care programs in each province typically includes goals such as: to support those individuals with chronic health needs to maintain health and quality of life; to complement, not replace, the support system of families and friends; to maintain independence and the ability of clients to live at home for as long as possible; and to maintain a system that is effective and efficient, and is fair to all regions and individuals.

Provinces have five basic requirements for long-term care eligibility: residency, health need, facility, assessment, and consent. The residency requirement entails proof of residence in a province or territory and a valid health insurance card for the jurisdiction where the services are being delivered. Need refers to health needs that cannot be met by family or from general community supports. For the facility requirement, the client must have a suitable home within which care may be provided or be admitted to a residential facility. An assessment of the client is performed to ascertain that the client requires care and to determine the client's ability to contribute to the cost of the care. Finally, the client must consent to treatment.

Within this overall framework, long-term care services are normally delivered by non-profit societies or for-profit organizations, under contract to the provincial Ministry of Health. In recent years, many provinces have established regional health authorities, which have responsibility for a full range of health services, including hospitals and long-term care.

Non-profit societies are required to meet certain conditions such as community representation, demonstrated commitment to quality of care, and an ability to deliver the care for which they are contracted. Almost all acute care hospitals in Canada are governed by non-profit societies or by regional authorities, but contracts to deliver home care or residential care can also be made with for-profit agencies. The latter contracts are normally made only with Ministry approval, especially when the Ministry provides the funding. In most cases, the for-profit agency would have to qualify through a public selection process. For-profit and non-profit agencies may also deliver privately funded care, provided they meet the Ministry standards.

In recent years, most provinces have made changes to strengthen community or regional governance systems. Under this system, funding for all health services in the region is prioritized, and programs are operated in a coordinated network of care by the regional authority. This regional approach has aimed to ensure that the client receives the most appropriate care, delivered by the most cost-effective part of the system, and has improved the delivery of care through greater integration of services to meet individual client needs.

ORGANIZATION OF THE DELIVERY SYSTEM AND RANGE OF SERVICES

Key Concepts

Long-term care is an umbrella concept used in Canada to describe a complex service delivery system comprising a full range of care and support for persons who have, or are at significant risk of having, progressive and/or chronic conditions, and who require services to meet their long-term functional needs. A number of more specific concepts within the overall concept of long-term care are consistently applied to achieve a coherent national approach to service delivery.

The four essential features of long-term care in Canada are that (1) the care will be long term; (2) it is an integrated program of care across various service components, that is, a service continuum; (3) it is a complex service delivery system, not a type of service; and (4) the efficiency and effectiveness of the system are based not only on the efficiency and effectiveness of each component, but also on the way that the service delivery system is structured.

The three components of long-term care service delivery systems are institutional care, community-based services, and home-based services, but the balance among these three components and the range of services within each vary from province to province, within an overall national framework that sets guidelines for access to care and complements the health care system. The following brief descriptions of service types highlight features of services that are distinctive to Canada and to particular provinces.

Continuing care has been used interchangeably with *long-term care* as a service concept, organizing framework (a continuum of services), and/or a division of government. Ontario, Prince Edward Island, and New Brunswick continue to use the term "long-term care," while other provinces use "continuing care" to describe the overall system and use the term "long-term care" to describe facility care.

Home care, for most provinces, refers to professional home-based services: nursing and rehabilitation. There are three distinct models of home care: maintenance and preventive, services that substitute for care in a long-term care facility, and services that substitute for acute care. This last model of acute care substitution is most distinct from the broader definitions of long-term care and continuing care.

While long-term care has been well established in Canada for many years, it is an evolving system that is changing in response to societal pressures, and change is proactive as well as reactive. As well as increasing diversity within the three broad service components, there is a trend towards services that link these elements, with services provided in one kind of setting reaching across to other settings to facilitate transfers of clients. It should also be noted that while the majority of long-term care service recipients are elderly, the system also serves disabled adults.

Residential Care Programs

The two main types of residential care services are chronic care hospitals or units within hospitals, and long-term care facilities, which are further divided into intermediate care facilities or facilities providing multiple levels of care that cover clients at intermediate and extended care levels.

Chronic care units and hospitals provide care to persons who, because of chronic illness and marked functional disability, require long-term institutional care but do not require all the resources of an acute, rehabilitation, or psychiatric hospital. Twenty-four hour coverage by professional nursing staff and on-call physician care is provided, as well as care by professional staff from a variety of other health and social specialties. Only people who have been appropriately assessed and who are under a physician's care are admitted. Care may be provided in designated Chronic Care Units in acute care hospitals (Extended Care Units, Discharge Planning Units, Chronic Behavior Disorder Units, etc.) or in freestanding Chronic Care Hospitals. Care requirements are typically 2.5 hours of professional nursing care per day or more. Only five provinces–British Columbia (BC), Northwest Territories, Manitoba, Quebec, and Newfoundland–include chronic care units under their long-term care programs.

Long-term care facilities are equivalent to nursing homes and lower levels of residential care in other countries and provide a protective and supportive environment for clients who can no longer live safely at home, together with varying levels of care services. Residents receive assistance with activities of daily living, 24-hour surveillance, assisted meal service, professional nursing care and/or supervision, including supervision with medication. Clients may have moderate to severe care needs that can no longer be safely or consistently met in the community. They may suffer from chronic diseases or from disabilities that reduce their independence and, generally, cannot be adequately cared for in their homes.

Home-Based Care Programs

The three main home-based services are homemaker, nursing, and allied health services, which are delivered to clients in their own homes. These services are generally similar to those in other countries, but some features warrant particular note.

Homemaker services are provided to clients who require non-professional (lay) personal assistance with care needs or with essential housekeeping tasks, and some specific nursing and rehabilitation tasks may also be delegated to homemakers.

Home care nursing provides comprehensive nursing care to people in their homes, generally by registered or psychiatric nurses, and includes coordination of nursing services and encourages clients and their families to be responsible for, and to actively participate in, their own care, thus promoting health education and self-care. Goals for home care nursing can be curative, rehabilitative, palliative, or supportive. Different provinces have different terminology for home care nursing: in New Brunswick, it is called home health care and in Newfoundland, community health nursing.

Community physiotherapy and occupational therapy services provide direct assessment, treatment, consulting, and preventive services to clients in their homes to monitor, rehabilitate, or augment function, or to relieve pain. Therapists may also arrange for necessary equipment to manage clients' physical disabilities and may train family members to assist clients appropriately. In Saskatchewan and New Brunswick, allied health services also include speech therapy, audiology, and respiratory therapy. *Equipment and supplies* are an adjunct to these services and a wide array of services operate for loan, purchase, or donation of equipment; examples are the Red Cross Loan Cupboard in British Columbia and New Brunswick, the Assistive Devices Program in Ontario, and the Aids to Daily Living Program in Alberta.

Community-Based Care Programs

There is some variation in the range of community-based care programs from province to province, around a core of common services.

Adult day care provides personal assistance, supervision, and an organized program of health, social, educational, and recreational activities in a supportive group setting, usually in the community, but may be provided within a residential care facility. The Yukon is the only jurisdiction in Canada with no adult day care program. In addition to adult day care, *respite services* are provided in the home or by alternate accommodation for the client in a residential setting.

Assessment and treatment centers or day hospitals are well-developed and provide short-term diagnostic, assessment, and treatment services in a special unit within an acute care hospital or other health facility. These centers provide intensive, short-term assessment services to ensure that persons with complex physical, mental, and social needs are correctly assessed, diagnosed, and treated. The objective of these centers is to assist the client to achieve, regain, and/or maintain an optimal level of functioning and independence. Centers may have beds for short-term inpatient assessment and treatment, a day hospital service, and/or an outreach capability that permits staff to assist clients who are in care facilities, in their own homes, or the homes of their families.

Palliative care services provide active, compassionate care to the terminally ill in their homes, in hospitals, or other health care facilities. The service is for individuals and their families where it has been determined that treatment to prolong life is no longer the primary objective.

Other services that are now widespread and standard parts of community-based care are *meals programs,* providing delivered meals to home or to centers, and *caregiver and other support groups* initiated from many sources such as community and institutional health services, friends of clients, and individuals having similar needs, to provide peer support and foster mutual aid, with some receiving government subsidies. *Volunteers* are utilized in addition to formal caregivers for a range of services such as friendly visiting, telephone assurance and monitoring, doing errands and shopping, and other social and recreational activities. In contrast to this array of services, *transportation services* are not part of the program in most provinces, although special assistance with transport is available through transit authorities and other agencies.

Finally, two kinds of congregate accommodations for frail aged and disabled people are viewed as part of community-based care in Canada because residents in these facilities are able to use all the same services as those living in their own homes. *Group homes or family care homes* enable persons with physical and/or mental disabilities to increase their level of independence through a pooling of resources. This type of care is particularly suited to disabled young adults who are working, enrolled in an educational program, or attending a sheltered workshop, but may also be provided to seniors. In Manitoba, there are various forms of this kind of housing–shared care, clustered care, block care, and supportive housing–but in other provinces this is not part of long-term care and is offered by other government departments such as Child and Family Services in Prince Edward Island, and Mental Health and Social Services in Saskatchewan.

Congregate living and assisted living residences are housing arrangements that offer amenities such as emergency response, social support, and shared meals. In some provinces, they also include the provision of supportive care to persons requiring minimal supervision and support with activities of daily living. Most of the congregate living residences are operated by organizations other than long-term care organizations. Examples of this program are Supportive Housing in British Columbia, Seniors Apartments in Alberta and New Brunswick, Assisted/Supportive Living in Saskatchewan and Ontario, and Enriched Housing Units in Nova Scotia.

SERVICE DELIVERY AT THE PROVINCIAL LEVEL

National consistency in access for clients is achieved through a substantial commonality in five features of provincial service delivery systems: access, assessment, classification, case management, and administration. At the same time, diversity in service delivery systems within provinces is increasing as provincial governments and service providers are developing innovative approaches to their particular needs and experimenting with alternative modes of service delivery.

Common Features

Single entry. Most provincial governments have, or are developing, a single entry system through community health centers and/or hospitals or health authorities. A single focal point or "one-stop shop" provides a consistent screening mechanism that ensures only those persons with demonstrated needs are admitted and that the appropriate level of care and other services are provided. Conversely, in systems without single entry points, people may not obtain care or the most appropriate level of care, because of a lack of knowledge about what is available to them.

In Ontario, Community Care Access Centers (CCACs) are responsible for entry to residential and home care nursing, but not for chronic hospital beds or community-based care. In British Columbia, Local Continuing Care or Long-Term Care Offices are responsible for entry to all residential care, including extended care units operated by acute care hospitals, and community- and home-based services. Prince Edward Island's Coordinated Single Entry System is another variant that operates through one call to one phone number; the caller is connected to the appropriate information or services across the long-term care system and can access a consistent and appropriate screening, the required needs and risk assessment, and referral to required services. All appropriate options for support and maintenance are reviewed and utilized through the Placement or Admission Committee, which prioritizes residential placement requests and expedites wait list management in each region. Requests and stated preferences from senior citizens are considered a priority.

Coordinated assessment and placement. Most provincial governments have their own standardized assessment tools for all long-term care clients, such as the Alberta Assessment and Placement Instrument. Ontario, Saskatchewan, Manitoba, Nova Scotia, British Columbia, and the Yukon have already, or are about to, implement one or more of the Resident Assessment Instrument/Minimum Data Set (RAI/MDS) series of assessment instruments. Nova Scotia has launched the Single Entry Agency–Levels of Eligibility and Need Evaluation System (SEA-LANES) in order to develop an eligibility algorithm for community and institutional services based on the MDS-Home Care (MDS-HC).

At the system level, consideration is given to whether or not clients can be cared for in the community as opposed to a facility. At a clinical level, the assessment and placement process maximizes the probability of providing the most appropriate services to meet clients' needs. Coordinated assessment allows for the collection of the same information for residential and community-based clients on admission to the overall care system.

Client care level classification. A number of provinces employ between two to seven levels of classification as a general means of grouping patients. However, many of these classification schemes have received little or no testing, and regional governments and service providers frequently question their validity.

Ontario and Saskatchewan have made the MDS 2.0 mandatory for chronic hospitals and nursing homes, respectively, with the primary intent of providing data that can be used to support funding. In part, this decision was based on the presence of a track record of scientific evidence supporting their use (see the article, "Long-Term Care Funding in Canada: A Policy Mosaic," for additional discussion).

Ongoing system-wide case management. Ongoing system-wide case management enables the provision of necessary services across the service components of the overall system and ensures that there is regular monitoring and review of client needs. In most of the provinces, case management will be transferred to staff of residential care facilities when a client is admitted, but in some provinces, including British Columbia and Nova Scotia, the long-term care case manager continues to coordinate services even after the client is admitted to a facility. When needs change, care plans are adjusted to ensure that there is a continuing match between the needs of the client and the care provided.

Single administration. Operational responsibility for health services, including long-term care, has been devolved to regional health boards or authorities. In most provinces, all long-term care services come under the responsibility of the same senior manager. There are several advantages in single administration. Funding can be more readily transferred between residential and community-based service in order to maximize system efficiencies, and policy issues are likely to be viewed in the context of the overall long-term care or continuing care system. The care staff also develops a sense of the overall long-term care system, the functions that each of the service components offers in the system, and the way that the needs of the client can best be met within the system. Finally, planning and resource allocation will be done on an overall system basis, rather than on a component-by-component basis.

Service Innovations

There has been considerable innovation in provincial service delivery systems in recent years, and the examples in Table 1 illustrate the diversity of these developments. In particular, examples are given of innovative services that link across the health and long-term care systems and that aim to offer more choices and services to clients, using technology to link clients' homes to a community center. These examples are typical of wider innovation in service systems, but they should not be taken as a complete or comprehensive account of all recent developments.

QUALITY MANAGEMENT

Long-term care quality management in all Canadian provinces is based on a set of common principles, but provinces vary in the range of mechanisms and methods used to pursue quality management and to promote best practice.

Quality Principles

The six principles of quality management are that care services should be:

- *Consumer focused:* Services are relevant to the client's needs and the client's right to provide input into service planning is recognized.
- *Wellness based:* Services are to preserve and promote "health" in its broadest sense: the overall well-being, dignity, and independence of clients and their families. Services should promote client independence and normalized living.

TABLE 1. Examples of Innovations in Provincial Long-Term Care Services

Substitutes for acute care	
British Columbia: Sub-acute care *Alberta:* Progressive care *Saskatchewan:* Convalescent care	• covers patients who have had surgery or hospital treatment and who need extra time to recover before going home. • support is given to patients requiring extended recuperation following acute care, primarily elderly, high-risk clients.
Quebec: Intensive functional rehabilitation services	• provides interventions for CVA, hip fracture, or complicated fracture, to promote optimum functional restoration. • services can be provided in both inpatient and outpatient settings. • duration of inpatient services is 2-3 months, outpatient services up to one year.
Substitutes for facility-based long-term care	
Alberta: Comprehensive home option integrated care of elderly (CHOICE)	• provides comprehensive coordinated program for seniors eligible for admission to the continuing care program but who continue to live in their own homes. • includes CHOICE day center with a full range of medical, social, and supportive services; transportation and homemaking services; 24-hour emergency response, and respite care.
Quebec: Outpatient psycho-geriatric services	• provides specialized services to assist, orient and treat people with psycho-geriatric problems. • information, training, and support for informal and formal caregivers are also provided.
Alberta: Mentally dysfunctional elderly unit	• provides assessment and transitional services designed to meet the unique needs of individuals experiencing irreversible dementia.
Yukon Territory: Outreach social workers for seniors	• provides services to street people and others who intentionally stay away from programs such as Home Care. • roles include advocacy, housing, and case management.
British Columbia: Quick response teams	• provide outpatient, inpatient, in home assessment, and referral to home care nursing, community physiotherapy, occupational therapy, and homemaker services on an emergency basis.
British Columbia: Choice in supports for independent living (CSIL)	• provides direct funding to clients or client group (societies). • client accepts all responsibilities of being a legal employer in hiring, firing, supervision, and payment of their homemaker.
Links between community-based and home-based care	
Saskatchewan: Security call	• regular scheduled telephone contact by contracted individuals to elderly, at-risk clients living in at home.
Ontario: Security checks or reassurance service	• provides isolated persons with regular contact to reassure them that help is available if and when needed. • may be provided by a person visiting the home, by telephone, or other means. • general security activity includes a short daily telephone call (less than 5 minutes) that checks the health and safety of the client.
Alberta: Lamplighter program	• trains people as "lamplighters" who watch for changes in a senior's condition that may signal a health or safety risk. • Senior's Health Line is advised, and follow-up is provided with the client concerned.
Ontario: Home maintenance and repair services	• provides or arranges for individual worker or company to undertake home maintenance or repair job. • work may be on a regular basis (e.g., yard maintenance and outside window washing), occasional or one time only (e.g., home repair or barrier free access modifications to improve quality of life).
Ontario: Foot care	• provides services such as trimming toe nails, monitoring the condition of feet, bathing and massaging feet by a person trained in basic or advanced foot care. • available to clients residing at home or attending adult day care center.
Ontario: Friendly visiting	• support service that matches a volunteer on a one-to-one basis to visit an isolated senior or physically disabled adult in his or her home on a regular basis. • volunteer may also do shopping for the client, take client shopping, to the bank, or to attend a social or cultural event.

- *Integrated:* Services are provided without interruption, and are coordinated across programs, practitioners, organizations and levels of service, and over time.
- *Accessible:* The individual is able to obtain services at the right place and at the right time, based on respective needs.
- *Appropriate:* The desired results are achieved with the most cost-effective use of resources.
- *Affordable:* Services are giving value for money and are provided within available resources, and funding mechanisms promote and reward efficiency and effectiveness.

Mechanisms and Methods to Ensure Quality of Services

A range of mechanisms is used in quality management, including use of professional standards, training requirements, human resource requirements, financial management requirements, organization process requirements, and mandated quality improvement process.

Standards for long-term care services adopted by Canadian provinces commonly address the following areas: administration, personnel, social environment, care services, and physical environment.

Legislation, regulations, policy, manuals and clinical practice guidelines are used to put standards into practice. Examples of legislation are the Nursing Homes Act and Home Care Regulations in Alberta, and the Continuing Care Act and the Hospital Act and Community Care Facility Act in British Columbia. Legislation is given effect through associated regulations, and policy and procedure manuals; examples of these are the *Long Term Care Facility Program Manual of Ontario* and the Service Provider Handbook, *Long Term Care Program,* in British Columbia. Saskatchewan also has extensive operational manuals: *Home Care Policy Manual, Home Care Policy Supplement, Home Care Nursing Manual, Home Care Information Systems Manual, Assessment and Care Coordination Binders,* and *Guidelines for Developing a Volunteer Program.* In Manitoba, there are numerous guidelines for delivering residential care services, including guidelines for infection control, for physicians' services in personal care homes, for adult day care, for use of restraints, and for maintenance of health records.

Committees have been established in a number of provinces to assist in the clarification, interpretation, and application of standards in long-term care facilities. In Ontario, there is a Long-Term Care Facility Program Standards Committee, with membership made up of representatives of the Health Ministry and service providers from the for-profit and not-for-profit sectors. There is also a Long-Term Care Facility Manual Advisory Support Group that reviews proposed changes and additions to standards specific to the *Long-Term Care Facility Program Manual.*

Ministry inspectors or compliance advisors have responsibility for monitoring and evaluating standards of care and services. They also investigate complaints and apply sanctions, such as withholding funding, stopping admissions, taking over the operation of a facility, revoking the license, and prosecution, as necessary.

Benchmarking is undertaken by making province-wide comparisons using data from the Minimum Data Set (MDS) or administrative data on service utilization (see the article "Long-Term Care Funding in Canada: A Policy Mosaic," for additional discussion).

Accreditation of the Canadian Council on Health Services Accreditation (CCHSA) is not mandatory in most provinces, but many service providers choose to take part in the national accreditation survey and to use CCHSA standards as their guide in developing their own quality management system.

Request for Proposal (RFP) is a funding mechanism that is also used to drive quality improvement. In Ontario, 90% of community-based care programs have been funded through an RFP process since April 1999. For-profit and not-for-profit agencies have an equal opportunity to compete for service contracts, and the quality principles of an RFP require each tendering agency continuously to improve the processes that enhance service delivery to the client, to have adequate human resources and financial management systems that function appropriately to meet stated goals and objectives, and to have a purpose and mission statement, a strategic plan, and a structure and functions that commit the organization to a client-focused approach to service delivery.

Other measures used for quality assurance in some provinces include a residents' bill of rights, internal agency quality management systems, and service agreements between the province and the provider agency.

Best Practice is promoted by provincial governments providing support for various demonstration projects. Best practice encourages the long-term care industry to look for initiatives in service programs and service delivery that combine best quality at best price. Two summary reports, "Innovations in Best Practice Models of Continuing Care for Seniors" and "Best Quality at the Best Price" have been published by the Federal/Provincial/Territorial Committee for the Ministers Responsible for Seniors (1988, 1999). Project initiatives were selected on the basis of six criteria: consumer/client focus, coordination and integration, efficiency and flexibility, program assessment and evaluation, education, and access. Although the process might not be scientifically rigorous, it does represent a national attempt to improve the effectiveness and efficiency of the system through inter-provincial/territorial benchmarking.

CHALLENGES FOR THE FUTURE

Pressures on Resources

After many years of relative stability, Canada's long-term care system is coming under increasing pressure from three main sources that are placing increased demands on limited resources, but neither public perceptions nor service providers seem willing to recognize and adjust to these pressures.

Increased demand is coming from changes within the care system. Complexity of needs is increasing as people are now being discharged from acute care hospitals sooner and so needing more complex post-hospital care for a longer period. Those with multiple chronic conditions are also living longer. As increasingly complex tasks are added to long-term care services, care is more costly to provide and more staff education is needed to provide the required knowledge and skills.

The interface between acute and long-term care is also changing, as there has been a push across Canada to provide more services in the community for non-acute care clients who were receiving services in acute care. More clients have been moved from acute care hospitals to the community, but funding for home- and community-based long-term care has not increased enough to meet this demand. The expectation that money would move from hospitals to the community with the change in location of service has not been realized, and it is questionable whether this transfer will ever take place because acute care hospitals will require more funds as they are treating patients with more complex conditions. The acuity and complexity of clients in the long-term care system have increased significantly, whereas the resources have remained more or less the same.

Public expectations have also grown and are often greater than programs are capable of meeting. Increased awareness and an increased seniors' lobby are putting pressure on the system for increased service delivery and the delivery of more complex services. Clients' perceptions of service "entitlement" and "need" make service reductions or program changes difficult to implement.

Clients are not the only ones to resist change; long-term care service providers also resist change. Many community-based services are being "forced" to form partnerships with new, often powerful, organizations and groups who have traditionally not viewed the long-term care sector as an equal partner.

Residential care can also be reluctant to give up control to the community-based sector and to resist the change of service focus from residential to the community level.

Continuing Strengths and Stresses

In terms of efficacy of financing, the Canadian system of long-term care certainly benefits from having one administrative system with one payer in each province, with cost-effectiveness decisions being taken across medical, hospital, long-term care, and other parts of the system. Long-term care programs generally contribute to the ability of the provinces to minimize expenditures on hospital care, allowing Canada to have relatively low rates of hospital beds per 1,000 population compared to other countries.

The long-term care system in Canada will, however, come under some stress during the next decade, as the population grows more elderly and as the cost of health care increases. Wait lists for long-term care services and beds are likely to increase, and alternative means of keeping elderly people at home and independent will continue to be sought. While the national framework for health and long-term care services will remain in place as this search continues, a recent report from Health Canada (1999) shows that provincial initiative will be a major source of change, and exchange of experiences among the provinces will become increasingly important in realizing the goals of national consistency in service delivery.

REFERENCES

Federal/Provincial/Territorial Committee of Officials (Seniors) for the Ministers Responsible for Seniors (1988). *Best Quality at the Best Price*. Ottawa: Division of Aging and Seniors, Health Canada.

Federal/Provincial/Territorial Committee of Officials (Seniors) for the Ministers Responsible for Seniors (1999). *Innovations in Best-Practice Models of Continuing Care for Seniors*. Ottawa: Division of Aging and Seniors, Health Canada.

Federal/Provincial/Territorial Subcommittee on Continuing Care (1991). *Future Directions in Continuing Care*. Ottawa: Health and Welfare Canada.

Health Canada (June 1999). *Home Care Development Provincial and Territorial Home Care Programs: A Synthesis for Canada*. Minister of Public Works and Government Services Canada.

Hollander, M. J., & Walker, E. (1998). *Report of Continuing Care–Organization and Terminology*. Ottawa: Division of Aging and Seniors, Health Canada.

Hollander, M. J., & Pallan, P. (1995). The British Columbia Continuing Care System: Service Delivery and Resource Planning. *Aging Clinical and Experimental Research*, 7(2).

Ministry of Health and Ministry Responsible for Seniors, The Province of British Columbia (1992). *Service Provider Policy Handbook–Long Term Care Program, Continuing Care Division.* Victoria, B.C.: Continuing Care Division, Ministry of Health.

National Advisory Council on Aging (1999). *Aging Vignettes–A Quick Portrait of Canadian Seniors.* Ottawa: Government of Canada.

Recent Developments in Aged Care Policy in Australia

Anna L. Howe, PhD

Consultant Gerontologist,
Immediate Past President, Australian Association of Gerontology

SUMMARY. A series of major reforms implemented through the mid 1980s sought to contain residential care and expand community care in Australia's long-term care system. While this goal has been maintained, a number of new policy initiatives followed the change of federal government in 1996. This article presents a systematic account of current policy objectives, implementation measures, and outcomes in three major policy areas: changing the balance between residential and community care, targeting in community care, and support for family caregivers. This analysis shows that while there have been shifts in emphasis from time to time, concerted policy efforts over the last 20 years have contained the growth of expenditure on long-term care and realized significant change in the service system. *[Article copies available for a fee from The Haworth Document Delivery Service: 1-800-HAWORTH. E-mail ad-*

Anna L. Howe, PhD, has held a range of research and teaching positions in Australian Universities, and from 1997-2000, she was President of the Australian Association of Gerontology. Dr. Howe's policy roles include four years as Director of the Federal Office for the Aged from 1989, and she has been an advisor to federal parliamentary committees and undertaken policy research for federal and state governments. Internationally, she has collaborated with the U.S. National Center on Health Statistics, and she has been a consultant to the UN, the WHO, and the World Bank.

Dr. Howe can be contacted at 123 Weston St., Brunswick, Victoria, Australia, 3056 (E-mail: anna.howe@bigpond.com).

[Haworth co-indexing entry note]: "Recent Developments in Aged Care Policy in Australia." Howe, Anna L. Co-published simultaneously in *Journal of Aging & Social Policy* (The Haworth Press, Inc.) Vol. 13, No. 2/3, 2001, pp. 101-116; and: *Long-Term Care in the 21st Century: Perspectives from Around the Asia-Pacific Rim* (ed: Iris Chi, Kalyani K. Mehta, and Anna L. Howe) The Haworth Press, Inc., 2001, pp. 101-116. Single or multiple copies of this article are available for a fee from The Haworth Document Delivery Service [1-800-HAWORTH, 9:00 a.m. - 5:00 p.m. (EST). E-mail address: getinfo@haworthpressinc.com].

101

KEYWORDS. Assessment, Australia, caregivers, community care, targeting, planning

THE POLICY CONTEXT

Recent Policy Directions

Since 1983, the consistent objective of aged care policy in Australia has been to move the balance of care away from residential care towards community care. Improved quality of care and equity of access have also been continuing policy goals.

Rather than being a continuum of care, the structure of Australia's aged care system is better seen as a set of building blocks, arranged in a pyramid as shown in Figure 1. The wide base of the pyramid represents the large number of frail older people living in the community with support from informal sources and relatively low inputs of formal services through the Home and Community Care Program (HACC). The middle range of support comprises increasing levels of formal community services mixed with a diversity of forms of supported accommodation. A variety of non-subsidized accommodation, ranging from serviced apartments in retirement villages to board and care homes, offers low levels of care services, together with federally funded hostels, which provide care to levels merging with the lower levels of nursing home care. The apex of the pyramid represents the highest levels of nursing home care.

If drawn on the basis of cost of services, the pyramid is inverted, and there are continuing upward cost pressures, including those associated with improving quality of care. The general goal of aged care policy can then be summarised as moving the balance of care towards lower cost services and maintaining the broad base of the service pyramid as a means of containing the high-cost services.

Since the change of federal government in 1996, policy has continued to build on the established aged care system, but new directions have been shaped by emerging problems identified in the field and by changed political philosophies. The 1996-97 federal budget signaled a move to rein in outlays by requiring those with capacity to pay to meet more of the costs of their care. These cost-containment policies have been pursued most vigorously in residential care and have been extensively reported elsewhere (Gibson, 1998; Howe,

FIGURE 1. The Aged Care Pyramid–Structure of the Australian Aged Care System

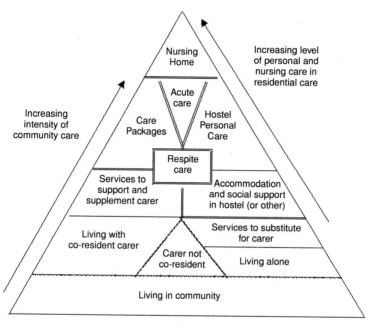

Access via Assessment Service

1997, 1998, 1999). Other initiatives to integrate the two previously separate hostel and nursing home levels of residential care through development of a single classification system for funding and implementation of a single quality assurance scheme are discussed in the next article, "Australian Approaches to Resident Classification and Quality Assurance in Residential Care." This article thus focuses on community care.

Detailed information on aged care programs in Australia can be found in *Australia's Welfare: Services and Assistance, 1999,* published by the Australian Institute of Health and Welfare (1999) and publications of the Commonwealth Department of Health and Aged Care (1999). [1]

Roles of Government

The roles of government in aged care in Australia are complex because each level of government–federal (or Commonwealth), state, and local–has different roles in policy development, funding, program administration, and service delivery, as summarised in Table 1. Relations between government and providers also reflect the differing involvement of the for-profit, not-for profit, and public sectors in residential and community care. There are also differences between the states and territories, in part because of different political parties being in office at any one time, and also because the role of local government in human services varies markedly among states.

The federal government has almost total responsibility for funding, planning, and monitoring residential care, but no role in direct service delivery. The major share of resources comes from general tax revenues, and the same federal benefits apply to all residents regardless of whether the provider is in the private-for-profit, not-for-profit, or state government sector. User fees now account for close to 30% of residential care funding. A large part of this revenue comes indirectly from the public purse because it is drawn from the Age Pension that 85% of residents receive in full or part. Australia's Age Pension is funded from general revenue and is income- and asset-tested. The private sector dominates the provision of nursing home care, with half the beds, followed by some 40% in the not-for-profit sector; the remainder are in the state government sector. Almost all hostel provision is in the not-for-profit sector.

In community care, state governments share responsibilities for policy development, funding, and program administration with the federal government. Government funding for HACC is cost-shared, with 48% of funds from the federal government, 32% from the states, and 20% from user fees. Almost 30% of HACC funds are allocated to agencies classified as state government providers, largely because of their statutory status under state legislation; the largest group of these agencies is composed of domiciliary nursing providers. Another 20% goes to local governments, but the largest share, half of all HACC funding, goes to the not-for-profit sector. While larger and longstanding community care providers are dominant, HACC stimulated the development of many smaller new community agencies, and more recently, not-for-profit residential care providers have been extending their role into community care. There is still only a small private-for-profit sector in HACC.

CHANGING THE BALANCE OF CARE

Policy Objectives

At the commencement of the Labor Government's Aged Care Reform Strategy in 1984-85, nursing home care dominated in terms of both provision and expenditure. Substantial changes were realised in the balance of care by

TABLE 1. Roles of Government and Non-Government Sectors in Aged Care

	Level of Government			Non-Government Sectors	
Residential Care	**Federal**	**State**	**Local**	**Not-for-profit**	**Private**
Policy development	Major	Minor	--	Major	Major
Funding[(a)]	Major	Minor	--	Minor	Moderate
Program admin.	Major	Minor	--	Minor	Minor
Service delivery	None	Minor	Minor	Major	Major
Community Care					
Policy development	Major	Major	Minor	Minor	--
Funding	Major	Moderate	Minor	Minor	--
Program admin.	Minor	Major	Moderate	Minor	--
Service delivery	None	Moderate	Major	Major	Minor

(a) Moderate funding role of private sector comes through capital construction.

the mid 1990s (Howe, 1998), but the pace of further shifts faltered due to the limited interest shown by either federal or state governments in expanding the cost-shared HACC program compared to initiating other small, short-term programs. Pressures in residential care also absorbed federal policy attention. At the same time, there has been increasing recognition of the role of community care in its own right, that is, supporting those with some level of handicap in the community who maintain their independence as far as possible, rather than just preventing admission to residential care.

Implementation Measures

Measures for changing the balance of care have been concerned with controlling overall demand for and supply of services, particularly residential care, and achieving a better match between client need and service provision.

Assessment for admission to residential care has been mandatory since the late 1980s, and a national network of Aged Care Assessment Teams (ACATs) is authorized to carry out the assessments. Assessment is not mandatory at the point of entry to community care, only for higher levels of services or care packages, as detailed below. Assessment is based on dependency and care needs; capacity to pay is taken into account only subsequently in determining the level of fees to be paid.

Needs-based planning processes apply to both residential care and community care. Planning the level and distribution of residential care is akin to the Unites States' Certificate of Need process. Development of nursing home beds and hostel places is governed by national ratios specified per 1000 population aged 70 and over; this population is deemed appropriate as fully 90% of individuals in residential care are aged 70 years and over (nursing homes providing care for younger people with severe disabilities were separated from the aged residential care program in 1985). The federal government issues an annual call for proposals to develop facilities in regions where provision is below the target ratios. In assessing the proposals that come forward, the government takes other factors into account, such as characteristics of the local population, the existing pattern of service provision, and the capacity of applicants to develop appropriate services. The planning process has been rigorously applied on a national basis for the last 15 years, and whatever other changes there have been in residential care policy, there has been no relaxation of control over levels of provision.

National Service Provision Targets (SPT) for the HACC program have developed more slowly, but have recently been defined in terms of the levels of service provision to be achieved as program outputs. In 1999, The Commonwealth Department of Health and Aged Care set up an Internet-based SPT system that enabled all HACC providers to access information on the target population and service provision targets for their local areas (*www.health.gov.au*). The SPT framework links service provision data for each region to the HACC client population, defined as those with moderate, severe, or profound handicaps. Following the definitions applied in surveys conducted by the Australian Bureau of Statistics, some 11% of the population aged 65 and over reported a moderate handicap–they have difficulty in performing ADL tasks. Fifteen percent reported severe or profound handicap–they sometimes or always need assistance (ABS, 1999). This target population differs from the population used in planning residential care; it is limited to the handicapped population, but includes all age groups, in accord with HACC's coverage of younger people with disabilities as well as the frail aged. Clients aged 65 years and over, however, account for 80% of HACC clients.

The HACC program covers a wide array of service types and includes a sub-program of Community Options Projects (COPs) that were introduced in the late 1980s. COPs provide case management and brokerage funds, which providers use to support clients with complex care needs in the community.

Outcomes

Whether described in terms of expenditure or the range of services available, the balance of care is now very different from that of the mid 1980s.

Expenditure trends as set out in Table 2 show the change in the balance of expenditure from the mid 1980s. Four main outcomes are evident:

TABLE 2. Trends in the Balance of Care: Expenditure on Aged Care, 1985-86 to 1997-98

Area of Expenditure	% of Aged Care Outlays				$m
	1985-86	1989-90	1993-94	1997-98[a]	1997-98
Nursing home	80.0	71.0	63.6	60.3	2847.3
Hostel	4.8	7.7	11.6	15.0	
Comm. Aged Care Packages	-	-	0.3	2.2	84.1
Home and Community Care	15.2	20.3	23.2	21.4	810.6
Assessment	<1.0	1.0	1.3	1.0	36.1
Total	100.0	100.0	100.0	100.0	3,778.1

Source: Derived from Australian Institute of Health and Welfare, *Australia's Welfare: Services and Assistance*, 1993, Table 5.14 and 1999, Table 6.23.
[a] Residential care was combined into a single program in 1997. Total residential care expenditure in 1997-98 reported at 75.4% of total outlays has been divided 80/20% between nursing homes and hostels, in line with the trend from 1993-94 to1996-97.

1. A marked shift away from residential care.
2. Within residential care, a shift from nursing home to hostel care.
3. Most of the shift in the balance of expenditure towards community care came about in the late 1980s and plateaued through the early 1990s; the share of total outlays going to HACC has been stable for some years now.
4. Change in the balance of expenditure towards community care is only being achieved through the substitution of Community Aged Care Packages for hostel places.

Service provisions show clear shifts in the balance of care, both within residential care and between residential and community care. The residential care planning process has made progress in reversing the 1985 balance of 60 nursing home beds and 40 hostel places per 1000 aged 70 years towards targets of 40 and 60 places, respectively, over a 20-year period, that is, by 2005. The persisting shortfall in hostel development saw the latter target modified in a number of steps from the early 1990s to reduce hostel places to 50 per 1000 and substitute 10 Community Aged Care Packages (CACPs) per 1000. Although CACPs remain part of the residential care planning ratios, they occupy an important position in the balance of care in relation to HACC. By mid 1999, total provision of 97 residential care places per 1000 aged population was divided among 47 nursing home beds, 41 hostel places, and 9 CACPs. This outcome demonstrates the effectiveness of the planning process in achieving the three main policy objectives of limiting growth of provision of nursing home care, directing new provision to areas of high need, and changing the balance among types of residential care.

The range of services funded under HACC has expanded considerably, and growth has been greater in newer service types. Data on service provision for 1993-94 to 1997-98 (AIHW, 1999) show changes in the balance of care within HACC as follows:

1. A relative reduction in home nursing in favor of personal care;
2. At the same time, an expansion of more intensive personal care ahead of basic home maker services and meals provision;
3. Substantial growth in respite care in day centers and in-home respite; and
4. Continuing low levels of home maintenance and modifications, notwithstanding these services being the area of greatest unmet need and serving very large numbers of clients at low unit cost.

TARGETING IN COMMUNITY CARE

Policy Objectives

Since the inception of HACC, there has been growing debate about how services should be targeted to clients with different levels of need, and as the early rapid growth of HACC stabilized, attention was directed to ensuring that resources went to "those most in need and who would benefit most."

The result was that smaller groups of clients came to absorb a disproportionate share of available service hours and, in turn, concerns emerged about the effects of reducing or withdrawing services from low-use clients. In 1995, the federal Department of Health and Aged Care commissioned a consultancy to investigate targeting strategies in HACC (Howe & Gray, 1999).

Implementation Measures

Unlike residential care, HACC had no formal arrangements for either assessment or classification of client needs. Assessment had not been made mandatory at the point of entry to the community care system because preserving open access was seen to be important in promoting early contact with the service system, and because the cost of full assessment would be disproportionate to the simple services that many clients required. Local agency staff were also well placed to make initial entry assessments and either undertake full assessments as necessary or refer clients to ACATs or other relevant agencies, for example, nursing services for assessment of skilled nursing needs. An informal "two-tier" system of assessment for community care has emerged, and policy has sought to develop a more consistent approach to formal assessment for all HACC clients with high needs (Lincoln Gerontology Centre, 1998). While HACC services clients at all levels of dependency, assessment is required only for those clients specifically seeking admission to COPs and CACPs.

Case management as a mechanism for resource allocation has been most formally implemented and funded through COPs and CACPs, and more recently, through a pilot program of nursing-home-level care packages. Case management practice is, however, found throughout the service system because the majority of CACPs and COPs providers are also HACC providers, and because most of the funds provided to these programs for brokerage are used to purchase services from HACC providers.

Outcomes

With no standard data collection in place at the time, the HACC targeting consultancy drew on client databases of seven major providers in five states, the largest of which served 30,000 clients annually, and the ACAT Minimum Data Base for 28,000 clients assessed in two states over a year. Relationships among client dependency, service use, and outcomes proved complex, but three general conclusions emerged.

First, the main function of HACC was confirmed as providing small amounts of service to a large number of clients. Resource allocation patterns in the seven major providers typically showed that about two thirds of clients received only low levels of service and absorbed only some 20% to 30% of service hours, and at the other extreme, a small group of 5% to 10% of clients consumed up to half the resources, with the balance taken by clients with intermediate levels of service use.

Second, the level of service use was not consistently related to client dependency. While no low-dependency clients used high levels of service, many high-dependency clients received only limited support from formal services. The mediating effect of support from family caregivers meant that level of service use was a poor indicator of dependency, and arbitrary decisions to withdraw service from clients using only low levels could have adverse outcomes since many relied greatly on those small service inputs.

The third and perhaps most telling finding came from the analysis of the relationship between use of services and the likelihood of recommendation for residential care on assessment by an ACAT. Clients who were already using a community service at the time of assessment were significantly less likely to be recommended for nursing home care than those using no services. This relationship was most evident for dependent clients who were most at risk of admission and thus had the greatest potential for risk to be reduced, whereas low-dependency clients had a very low risk of admission anyway. Against the apparent beneficial effect of initial service support, there appeared to be diminishing returns to further service inputs.

These findings suggest that community care in Australia plays a similarly important part in maintaining high-dependency clients in the community as reported in the United States by Liu, Manton, and Aragon (2000), but that there is a wider coverage of clients at lower levels of dependency who typically use low levels of service and consume a very small share of total community care resources. Further, the findings point to the need to moderate targeting strategies that concentrate even more resources on a small group of clients using high levels of services and the need to maintain provision of basic services to a wider population. The main priority identified was the provision of initial services to high-dependency clients who were not using any services at the time of assessment. Not only were these initial services potentially more effective in forestalling admission, but the absolute size of this group of clients was much larger than the small number using multiple services, and many were able to remain in the community only because of very substantial support from informal caregivers. Providing some initial service to high-dependency clients who have so far not received any services is also arguably more equitable than giving additional resources to those already receiving high levels of support. The implications for the balance of care to be provided by community services are that a spread of services across a larger number of clients and across a range of dependency levels may achieve more beneficial outcomes overall than targeting increasingly high levels of service on a small group of clients, especially when this concentration comes at the cost of withdrawal of services from others.

A final consideration in the targeting debate is that attempts to demonstrate the benefits of case management for highly dependent clients have been no more successful in Australia than in the United States. While case management is well accepted by providers and clients, the findings of evaluations of case-managed programs in Australia are at best ambivalent regarding outcomes (see, for example, Charlton et al., 1992; Gray et al., 1995; Wells, Swerissen, & Kendig, 1999; Kendig et al., 1999). As case management *per se* incurs a cost, it has been reserved for a select group of clients with complex needs and requiring coordination of multiple services. There were only some 14,000 CACPs and some 5,000 frail aged COPs clients in 1999 compared to over 400,000 frail aged clients receiving HACC services over a year. However, as access to case-managed care packages seems set to grow ahead of access to basic HACC services, take-up will likely extend to increasingly less dependent clients. The potential perverse outcome for the balance of care will be an upward gravitation to using higher than necessary levels of resources because of restricted access to the basic, necessary level of care.

SUPPORT FOR INFORMAL CAREGIVERS

Policy Objectives

With the establishment of the HACC Program in 1984, caregivers were recognized as clients in their own right, and a range of services was developed to assist carers in recognition of their contributions to supporting frail aged people as well as younger people with disabilities. In Australia, the term "carers" is used for informal caregivers, mainly family members; paid carers in formal services are referred to as "staff" or "care workers."

Three factors that have contributed to strengthening care policy warrant brief comment. First, beyond recognition of the value of carer contributions *per se,* the provision of assistance to family carers was seen as having the capacity to delay entry to residential care and thereby moderate demand, and to do so in a cost-effective manner.

Second, support provided to carers' representative organisations through HACC saw them grow in influence and gain a greater voice in policy debates. Partly in response to this increased political profile, a variety of short-term carers' initiatives has been taken outside the HACC program by both the federal and state governments, and carer support is now identified as a third strand in the long-term care system, alongside residential and community care. A National Agenda for Carers was developed in 1996 (Department of Human Services and Health, 1996). Implementation has proceeded steadily since (Perring, 2000), and several states have developed or are in the process of developing carer strategies.

Third, and more generally, support for family carers reflects community norms of intergenerational exchange and reciprocity, which have been widely reported in studies of caregiving in Australia (Schofield, 1998). These norms remain strong in the Australian community and are endorsed by a central focus on families in federal government social policy. Support for family caregivers sits comfortably within the ambit of its approach to social policy, based on mutual obligation between the state and other sectors, including individuals and families.

Implementation Measures

The development of integrated carer support strategies has drawn on four main channels of funding and service provision.

HACC services are the foundation of care support; either directly or by assisting the person for whom they care, and HACC is thus the main source of carer support services.

Federal and state initiatives have been taken outside HACC to expand carer support, focusing mainly on information and advisory services to improve access to respite care through various Carers' Packages and Carers' Strategies. The National Respite for Carers initiative has provided funding to expand all kinds of respite services and Carer Resource Centers in each state, and a Carelink network is being developed to provide a single point of telephone access to information in all regions.

Access to residential respite care has been facilitated through a range of measures, including payment of a specific respite benefit to providers and booking services run by ACATs, in addition to the respite access measures noted above.

Two cash benefits are available to carers of handicapped individuals of all ages. The Carer Payment is part of the social security system and provides income support to caregivers who are unable to work because of their caring responsibilities. The payment is at the same level as other income support payments and subject to the same means tests. It is paid by exception to eligible caregivers who do not qualify for other income support payments; the majority of older people who are caregivers and who quality for income support thus receive it via the Age Pension rather than the Carer Payment. The Carer Allowance is paid to full-time caregivers, on a non-means tested basis, to assist with the costs of caregiving, where the person cared for would otherwise be in residential care. Set at a much lower rate than the Carer Payment, the Carer Allowance is paid in recognition of the carer's role; it is not regarded as an income support payment or as a salary for the work of providing care. Caregivers who receive the Carer Payment can also receive the Carer Allowance.

Outcomes

Three indicators of the interaction between carer policy and carer roles can be given. First, in response to several reports of respite being the service that carers identified as their greatest need, there has been substantial growth of all forms of respite care. In residential care, for example, respite admissions grew from 5% of admissions in 1990 to over 25% by the late 1990s, and there has also been steady growth in respite admission to hostels. In HACC, hours of respite care in day centers and in-home respite have grown ahead of other service types.

Second, a number of evaluation studies have pointed to the effect of the presence of a carer on moderating levels of service use (see, for example, Kendig et al., 1992; Mathur, Evans, & Gibson, 1997). In community care, clients with carers use fewer services and remain in the community with higher levels of dependency than those without carers. In residential care, the importance of carers is seen in the over-representation of those previously living alone.

Third, an overview of the balance of care coming from informal and formal sources is given by the findings of the ABS Survey of Disability, Ageing and Carers (Australian Bureau of Statistics, 1999). Focusing on the 30% of the older population defined as having moderate, severe, or profound activity restrictions as above,

- just under one third were supported by informal care only,
- just over a third received a mix of formal services and support from informal caregivers,
- some 13% were in the community with support from formal services only,
- some 16% were in residential care, mostly federally subsidised nursing homes and hostels, and
- a small group, about 3%, remained in the community without any support.

The mix of informal and formal support found in Australia cannot be easily compared to the kinds of support in other countries. Focusing only on those in the community, the mix noted above indicates that in Australia, some 57% of those aged 70 and over with at least a moderate level of handicap had access to some community care, either as a sole means of assistance or as an adjunct to informal support. Data for 1994 for the United States show that the proportion of those aged 65 and over receiving help from paid sources only or a mix of paid and informal helpers, as compared to informal helpers only, reached this level only for the most dependent, those with five or more ADLs, and tapered down to 35% for those with only one ADL (Liu, Manton, & Aragon, 2000). Interpretation of these data must be cautious due to differences in the age groups covered and differences in the measurement of dependency and range of dependencies included. However, consistent with the pattern noted above, community care appears to offer wider coverage at lower levels of dependency in Australia and comparable coverage at higher levels of dependency, although with less intensity of service.

PROSPECTS FOR CONTINUING CHANGE IN THE BALANCE OF CARE

Australia's experience over the last 20 years suggests that population aging does not necessarily mean an increase in social outlays. While the population aged 65 years and over in Australia grew by 50% from 1981 to 1996, the proportion of aged increased only from 10% to 12% of the population. GDP (Gross Domestic Product) has also grown steadily through that time, and the share of GDP spent on social outlays for the aged, including aged care, health, and income support, has remained remarkably stable at about 5% (Choi, 1998). This outcome has been realized through purposeful policy decisions that have shaped programs and services to meet changing needs, taking account of prevailing macro-economic conditions and in a manner consistent with community values. With continuing concerted effort, it seems reasonable that similar outcomes can be realized in future.

Against this overall stability, the shift of the balance of care towards community has progressed more unevenly. The expansion of community care through the late 1980s came from additional resources being committed to community care rather than from savings in residential care, but this growth stalled in more recent years. While the level of provision of residential care overall has been contained, each place has become relatively more costly; this escalation was especially pronounced in the late 1990s when the nexus between levels of provision of hostel and nursing home places and levels of benefits was removed and upwards classification of a substantial proportion of hostel residents ensued.

The impact of this increase on government outlays has been moderated first by the imposition of increased user charges, but the increase in the cost of residential care to the community was substantial. Second, the expansion of hostel places has persistently fallen below the target ratios set, and while releasing funds from residential care to be transferred to community care packages, the packages have been funded at a rate equivalent to the lowest level of care benefit. However, rather than policy leading the transfer of resources to community care by reducing the ratio for hostel provision, the decision was made only after the hostel shortfall had been evident for some years, with the contributing factors including provider uncertainty in a climate of changing capital funding and consumer access to a wider market of retirement accommodations. The federal government's decision to channel the savings from hostels into care packages has enabled it to maintain the place of community care in the overall balance of care without increasing its commitments to HACC, and somewhat paradoxically, has relieved state governments of having to increase their cost-shared contribution to HACC.

The early expansion of HACC and the more recent growth in packages has no doubt provided alternatives to residential care, but the relationship is far from a simple trade-off between the two modes of care. Recognition of the multiplicity of factors underlying the shift in the balance of care is a salutary reminder that, while aged care policy in Australia has been characterized by a considerable level of rational planning, drawing on extensive empirical data and findings from service monitoring, evaluations, and reviews, policy-making is essentially a political process. The involvement of three levels of government, the private sector, the traditional voluntary sector and newer community organizations, professional bodies, and consumer groups gives rise to a diversity of interest groups, and at times competing interests, in aged care policy development in Australia. The balance of care reflects the balance of power among these interest groups, and changes in the balance of power are as important in determining the balance of care as any array of rational policy measures.

NOTE

1. The Commonwealth Department of Health and Aged Care has undergone a series of name changes as its functions have changed from time to time, and also appears as the Department of Human Services and Health, and the Department of Health, Housing and Community Services. For information on aged care programs, see *www.health. gov.au*

REFERENCES

Aged and Community Care Division and Office of Disability, Department of Human Services and Health (1996). Towards a national agenda for carers: Workshop papers. *Aged and Community Care Service Development and Evaluation Reports.* No. 22. Canberra: Australian Government Printing Service.

Australian Bureau of Statistics (ABS) (1999). *Disability, Aging and Carers: Summary of Findings.* ABS Catalogue No. 4430.0.

Australian Institute of Health and Welfare (AIHW) (1999). *Australia's Welfare 1999: Services and Assistance.* Canberra: Australian Government Publishing Service. See also *www.aihw.gov.au*

Australian Institute of Health and Welfare (1993). *Australia's Welfare 1993: Services and Assistance.* Canberra: Australian Government Publishing Service.

Bishop, B. (Minister for Aged Care) (1999a). *The National Strategy for an Ageing Australia: Background Paper.* Canberra: AusInfo.

Charlton, F., Arch, M., Carter, M., Humphries, S., & Todd, M. (1992). Ballarat and Bendigo Linkages Study: A comparison of outcomes for geriatric assessment clients. *Aged and Community Care Service Development and Evaluation Reports.* No. 5. Canberra: Australian Government Printing Service.

Choi, C. Y. (1998). Government health and welfare expenditure on older Australians. *Welfare Division Working Paper.* No. 20. Canberra: Australian Institute of Health and Welfare.

Department of Health and Aged Care (1998). *Two-Year Review of Aged Care Reforms: Issues Paper.* Canberra: Department of Health and Aged Care.

Department of Human Services and Health (1996). Towards a national agenda for carers. *Aged and Community Care Service Development and Evaluation Reports.* No. 22. Canberra: Australian Government Printing Service.

Gibson, D. M. (1998). *Aged Care: Old Policies, New Problems.* Cambridge: Cambridge University Press.

Gray, L., Appleby, N., Farish, S., & Sullivan, M. (1995). *Bundoora Community Care Project.* Melbourne: Centre for Applied Gerontology, Bundoora Extended Care Centre.

Hindle, D. (1998). Classifying the care needs and services received by HACC clients. *Aged and Community Care Service Development and Evaluation Reports.* No. 33. Canberra: Australian Government Printing Service.

Howe, A. L. (2000). Rearranging the compartments: The financing and delivery of care for Australia's elderly. *Health Affairs, 19*(3): 57-71.

Howe, A. L. (1999). Future directions for residential care. *Australasian Journal on Ageing, 18*: 12-18.

Howe, A. L. (1998). The economics of aged care: Achieving quality and containing costs. In G. Mooney & R. Scotton (Eds.), *Economics and Australian Health Policy.* Sydney: Allen & Unwin.

Howe, A. L. (1997). The aged care reform strategy: A decade of changing momentum and margins for reform. In A. Borowski, S. Encel, & E. Ozanne (Eds.), *Ageing and Social Policy in Australia.* Sydney: Longman Cheshire.

Howe, A. L., & Gray, L. (1999). Targeting in the home and community care program. *Aged and Community Care Service Development and Evaluation Reports.* No. 37. Canberra: Department of Health and Aged Care.

Kendig, H., McVicar G., Reynolds, A., & O'Brien, A. (1992). *Victorian Linkages Project Evaluation.* Canberra: Department of Health, Housing, and Community Services and Victorian Department of Human Services.

Kendig, H., Wells, Y., Swerissen, H., & Reynolds, A. (1999). Costs of community care services for individuals with complex needs. *Australasian Journal on Ageing, 18*: 86-92.

Lincoln Gerontology Centre (1998). National framework for comprehensive assessment of the HACC Program. *Aged and Community Care Service Development and Evaluation Reports.* No. 34. Canberra: Australian Government Publishing Service.

Liu, K., Manton, K. G., & Aragon, C. (2000). Changes in home care use by disabled elderly persons: 1982-1994. *Journal of Gerontology, 55B*: S245-53.

Mathur, S., Evans, A., & Gibson, D. (1997). Community aged care packages: How do they compare? *Aged and Community Care Service Development and Evaluation Reports.* No. 32. Canberra: Australian Institute of Health and Welfare and Department of Health and Family Services.

Perring, R. (2000) Commonwealth government support for carers with particular reference to information services and respite provision: The Australian perspective. Paper presented at 2nd International Conference on Caring, Brisbane.

Schofield, H. (Ed.). (1998). *Family Caregivers: Disability, Illness and Ageing.* Sydney: Allen & Unwin.

Wells, Y., Swerissen, H., & Kendig, H. (1999). Client outcomes in case managed care: Who benefits most? *Australasian Journal on Ageing, 18*: 79-85.

Australian Approaches
to Resident Classification
and Quality Assurance in Residential Care

Richard C. Rosewarne, PhD

Director, Applied Aged Care Solutions

SUMMARY. This paper begins with an account of the structure of Australia's residential long-term care program, which was divided into two distinct levels of hostel and nursing home care until 1997. In response to changed policy objectives, a number of measures were then taken to create an integrated residential care system. The main measures were the development of a single scale for classification of resident care need and associated funding to replace two previous separate scales, and the implementation of a new quality assurance system, which included new standards for buildings as well as revised standards for care. I give ac-

---

Dr. Richard C. Rosewarne is Director of Applied Aged Care Solutions. He is a registered psychologist and has worked in the Aged Care field for the past 18 years as a senior research fellow and more recently as director of a consulting company. He has extensive experience in the general aged care and aged psychiatry sectors with clinical research projects, strategic information collection, and analysis and design of large-scale projects. He also has spent considerable time working with staff in aged care facilities and has had hands-on clinical experience with older people with dementia and their carers. He has advanced skills with research and survey project methodology and knowledge and experience with information systems and database management and analysis.

Dr. Rosewarne can be contacted at Applied Aged Care Solutions Pty Ltd., 14 Nathan Rd., Eltham, 3095, Melbourne, Australia (E-mail: Richard.Rosewarne@AgedCareSolutions. com) or from the company web site (www.Aged CareSolutions.com).

[Haworth co-indexing entry note]: "Australian Approaches to Resident Classification and Quality Assurance in Residential Care." Rosewarne, Richard C. Co-published simultaneously in *Journal of Aging & Social Policy* (The Haworth Press, Inc.) Vol. 13, No. 2/3, 2001, pp. 117-135; and: *Long-Term Care in the 21st Century: Perspectives from Around the Asia-Pacific Rim* (ed: Iris Chi, Kalyani K. Mehta, and Anna L. Howe) The Haworth Press, Inc., 2001, pp. 117-135. Single or multiple copies of this article are available for a fee from The Haworth Document Delivery Service [1-800-HAWORTH, 9:00 a.m. - 5:00 p.m. (EST). E-mail address: getinfo@haworthpressinc.com].

117

counts of these measures and the extent to which they have achieved their intended outcomes before proposing some further developments that could see closer links among pre-admission assessment, resident classification, and quality assurance. *[Article copies available for a fee from The Haworth Document Delivery Service: 1-800-HAWORTH. E-mail address: <getinfo@haworthpressinc.com> Website: <http://www.HaworthPress.com> © 2001 by The Haworth Press, Inc. All rights reserved.]*

KEYWORDS. Australia, residential care, assessment, resident classification, quality of care, certification, accreditation

ORGANIZATION OF SERVICE DELIVERY

Use of Residential Care

As of mid 1997, a total of 126,897 residents aged 65 years and over were accommodated in the 139,058 beds in federally funded nursing homes and hostels in Australia; of the small number of residents below age 65, most were aged over 50. Just 3.1% of the population aged 65 and over were in nursing homes and 2.6% in hostels (AIHW, 1998a, 1998b). The proportion of the aged population in nursing homes is in the lower range for OECD countries, and the total proportion in both forms of residential care is comparable to most western countries but higher than in the rapidly aging countries of Asia. The overall level of residential care has been stable for some years now, the outcome of sustained efforts to contain the use of residential care.

While only a small minority of all older people is in residential care at any one time, a larger number spend some time in care over their lifetimes. Over the year 1996-97, there were a total of 88,271 admissions to residential care; these were divided between 32,252 admissions to nursing homes for permanent care and 12,612 for respite care; and 19,900 admissions to hostels for permanent care and 23,507 for respite care. Life table modeling by the Australian Institute of Health and Welfare has further shown that an individual aged 65 years of age has a 35% chance of entering a nursing home and a 25% chance of entering a hostel in his or her remaining lifetime (AIHW, 1997). This finding is important because it emphasizes that use of some form of residential care will be a reality for a large proportion of the population in the later stages in their lives.

Types of Facilities and Care Services

There are two types of facilities in the formal residential care program in Australia: 1,470 nursing homes provide 74,400 beds, and 1,497 hostels provide 63,145 beds. Nursing homes deliver 24-hour skilled nursing care and accommodation services to highly dependent residents. Half of these residents remain in care for stays of less than 12 months. National data show that around 40% of people admitted to nursing homes were already living in a hostel or some other kind of supported care or congregate housing prior to admission, and more significantly, fully 63% of admissions followed an episode in an acute hospital (AIHW, 1998a).

Hostels provide accommodation services, social support, and personal care by way of assistance with tasks of daily living, such as dressing and mobility. Models of care are primarily social in nature, and stays in hostels are considerably longer than nursing home care, with average stays of around four years. Again in contrast to the nursing home admission profile, close to 80% of hostel residents were living in the community immediately prior to admission, with the majority of the others living in various forms of congregate housing or specialized retirement accommodation (AIHW, 1998b).

The level and nature of care provided in hostels, including modified environments, is similar to assisted living facilities in the United States. Almost all hostel provision is in the not-for-profit sector. While some hostels are co-located with nursing homes and/or more independent forms of accommodation in developments providing several levels of care, many are operated separately from any other levels of care. Single-level provision is even more common for nursing homes; half of all nursing home beds are in the for-profit sector, and very few of these operate in conjunction with other levels of care. The major part of overall nursing home provision is thus in facilities that are not associated with hostels.

Since October 1997, several measures have been taken to bring the planning, administration, and funding of nursing homes and hostels together in an integrated system. Nursing homes and hostels have been re-designated as high-care and low-care facilities, respectively, and while most will continue to specialize in high care or low care, some have taken the opportunity to offer the full range of care services to allow residents to remain in the one facility as their care needs increase. This approach, called "aging in place," is designed to promote delivery of support services where the person is, rather than the person having to move to another facility as his or her needs change. The practicalities of aging in place have been the subject of some debate, and integration has especially raised issues about requirements for nursing staff in hostels because, until 1997, hostels were not required to provide 24-hour nursing care, although many did have nurses on their staffs. Hostels that opt for aging in place are now required to have registered nursing staff, while those taking only low-care residents can either employ nursing staff or engage visiting nursing services as required.

Mandatory Pre-Admission Assessment

A national network of Aged Care Assessment Teams (ACATs) has been operating since the mid 1980s, and ACATs have a central role in ensuring equity of access and sustainability for residential and community services. Older people cannot enter a nursing home or hostel or receive an intensive package of community care services without an ACAT assessment.

ACATs are usually based in public hospitals and undertake multidisciplinary assessments of the medical, psychological, and social care needs of older people living in the community and in aged care facilities. Where available, family caregivers are involved in the assessment. Outcomes of assessments most often result in a recommendation to remain in the community with supports from the Home and Community Care Program (HACC) or a care package, or referral to rehabilitation services. Only some 20% of assessments result in a recommendation for admission to residential care, and the ACAT also recommends whether hostel or nursing home care is appropriate.

ACATs are independent from providers, and ACAT performance is monitored by the federal Department of Health and Aged Care through regular evaluation that includes reporting of a Minimum Data Set. The ACATs compile a detailed profile of each client's dependency at the time of assessment, but this information is not at present used in subsequent funding classification of those who are admitted to residential care or in monitoring of quality of care.

The processes of ACAT assessment, resident classification, and quality assurance are summarized in Figure 1. While there is some interaction among those involved in each of these processes in the day-to-day delivery of long-term residential care, the accounts of the classification and quality assurance processes that follow show that while recent developments have strengthened the operation of these processes, they operate largely independently. The development of formal links among the processes, especially by way of information transfers and data linking, is a means for fostering further improvements in all parts of the system and so promoting quality of care throughout.

RESIDENT CLASSIFICATION

History

Various systems of classification of residents in long-term care facilities have provided a basis for national funding for over 30 years in Australia. The current system has evolved considerably since the first two-tier classification of nursing home residents into "ordinary care" and "extensive care" was intro-

FIGURE 1. Summary of Pre-Admission Assessment, Resident Classification, and Quality Assurance Processes in Residential Care in Australia

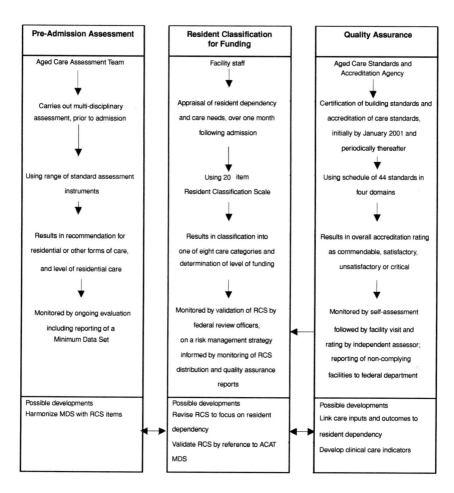

duced in 1969, some six years after the commencement of federal funding for nursing home care. This basic scheme rested on only superficial assessment of care needs by the facility staff, and in the absence of pre-admission screening, created a perverse incentive for facilities to admit the least dependent resident for whom the extensive care benefit could be claimed, although facilities did not have to meet extra nursing care requirements. There was no effective scrutiny of benefit claims. Notwithstanding these problems, the ordinary/extensive care classification remained essentially unchanged until 1988 when the Resident Classification Instrument (RCI) was introduced in nursing homes.

The RCI provided funding for five categories of nursing home residents using a 14-item scale, with rating at four levels of dependency on each item. The RCI also included an "overall service need" item as a dependent variable, and the scale was calibrated and the items weighted via factor analytic and regression methods. The standard weights showed the relative importance of each item to the overall service need. As an additive or continuous index, the RCI allowed a score to be calculated for every individual resident by taking the rating on each item, applying the standard weight, and then summing the weighted ratings on all 14 items. The distribution of scores obtained in large-scale trials conducted during the development of the RCI was then divided into five categories, with cut-off points and levels of funding set by the federal Department so as to contain overall expenditure within the existing budget. In providing a funding tool through which levels of reimbursement are related to residents' dependency and care needs, the RCI paralleled the implementation of Resource Utilization Groups (RUGs) in the United States, except that the Australian system of classification was implemented nationally.

Classification of hostel residents followed a similar history. Federal funding for construction of hostels commenced under the Aged Persons' Homes Act in 1954, but a two-tiered system of recurrent funding for care was not implemented until 1969 when the Personal Care Subsidy was introduced for residents requiring personal care. Other residents requiring only "hostel care" paid fees to cover board and lodging; the level of fees that could be charged was subsequently controlled by linking to the Age Pension to protect access for those on low incomes.

Partly in response to the implementation of the RCI in nursing homes and to promote the provision of additional programs for residents with dementia, this simple system of personal care and hostel care was replaced with an expanded scale in 1992. The 16-item Personal Care Assessment Instrument (PCAI) with 12-ADL related questions and four behavior questions was used to determine three levels of subsidy–Personal Care High, Medium, and Low–and residents not requiring personal care were classified in a fourth category, Hostel Care Only. The PCAI item weightings were determined in a similar way as for the RCI.

Both the RCI and PCAI had much in common with other dependency assessments in use in other countries, with items in the scales covering care needs in ADLs such as mobility, continence, bathing, and dressing, and also covered cognitive ability, behavior, and nursing treatments and procedures. However, at the time the PCAI was introduced, the option of extending the RCI to hostels was not considered. Rather than being an extension of nursing homes providing a lower level of much the same kind of care, hostels were seen as providing a distinctly different model of care to residents who required a range of social supports and personal care but not ongoing nursing care from registered nurses.

Pressures for Change

Through the mid 1990s, a number of pressures that had emerged in the classification and funding systems precipitated a review of the two separate classification systems. The need for change was also prompted by the need to integrate the two separate systems to bring them into line with the wider restructuring of residential care that followed the change of federal government in early 1996.

First, changes were evident in the dependency profile of the residential care population, particularly in hostels. Over the decade to the mid 1990s, the aged population, especially the very old, had increased substantially while the number of nursing home beds was relatively unchanged, and the number of hostel beds increased considerably. The level of dependency of residents in nursing homes increased as those with lower levels of dependency were diverted to hostels, in turn raising the dependency profile of hostels. Expanded community care could also now support some of those at the lower levels of personal care who would previously have been supported in hostels. The classification scales had thus been calibrated on resident populations that were markedly different from the current populations. Dementia care was especially a much more important issue than was the case 10 years previously when the RCI was introduced, and although the PCAI aimed to address dementia care, it was only partly successful in doing so.

Second, there was considerable criticism of the structure of both scales from care staff and service providers regarding biases within the scales. In particular, it was considered that dementia care and behavioral support needs were not clearly or sufficiently acknowledged in the RCI and that funding was instead too strongly linked to ADL dependency to the exclusion of other care needs. This was an artifact of the method used to calibrate the RCI. As the item weightings had been based exclusively on the first principal component, which related only to physical care needs, it was argued that items strongly related to other independent factors covering behavioral care needs, sensory impairments, and specialized nursing requirements were under-weighted, even though dependencies in these areas contributed to ADL dependency. Residents scoring highly on items with low weightings received considerably less funding than staff believed appropriate.

Third, service providers were strongly of the opinion that linking funding to dependency was a problem. They argued that there was no incentive for staff to focus on helping residents retain as much independent functioning as possible because funding was always linked to dependency, not staff successes with improving resident functioning. Staff and providers believed this encouraged a "do it for them" culture, as it often took longer to guide residents through their personal care routines than to assist them directly.

Finally, there was contention about the way in which the continuum of RCI scores was divided into categories and how funding levels were determined. The federal department overseeing the development of the RCS had determined the cut-points for the bands by reference to the available funding pool, and notwithstanding insistence that the RCI was a measure of relative rather than absolute care needs, providers believed that the funding made available for each category had little relationship to the actual cost of care even in a relative sense.

The options for developing a new classification system were (1) to remove redundant questions, add new questions to fill assessment gaps, and re-weight the existing scales, or (2) to develop a completely new, single classification covering both hostels and nursing homes. The government decided on the second option primarily because this approach accorded with the wider policy goal of integrating hostels and nursing homes into a single system of residential care, within which aging in place could also be promoted. In this case, a classification system had to be developed that would correctly locate residents whose needs varied from low levels of personal care, through those with mild to severe dementia, to those with intensive nursing care needs, on a nationally consistent scale.

Development of the Resident Classification Scale

The development of the new classification scale was the subject of detailed technical investigation reviews, consultations with providers, large-scale field trials, and extensive statistical analysis, and these activities have been well documented (Hindle, 1996; Rhys Hearn, 1997).

The first step was the selection of resident characteristics that were highly related to the cost of care. This selection was made by canvassing staff in aged care facilities about resident characteristics they felt were most strongly related to the cost of care and examination of existing information on cost-related resident characteristics. A cost/time variable was also developed from a study that examined staff costs, staff time spent on resident care, and the cost of consumables such as dressings, continence products, etc. Relationships between the time/cost variable and data on activities of daily living, behavioral care, nursing care, and social needs were then analyzed to determine which of these data items were most highly related to the "cost" of care.

Once the set of candidate predictor items was developed, a draft scale was trialled in a survey of some 20,000 residents. Extensive analyses of the data collected in these trials informed decisions about key aspects of the new scale, namely:

1. Whether an additive multiple regression model (like the old RCI) or a branching model (a regression tree like RUGs or DRGs) should be used to determine level or membership of a payment class;
2. Whether bands or funding groups should be used if an additive model was selected or whether continuously varying scores would be allowed; and
3. How the payment rate per band/group would be determined.

It was decided that an additive approach was most appropriate on both methodological and practical grounds. An additive model is seen as a better predictor of cost where a continuous distribution is used to determine payment classes. Whereas patients in acute care settings differ in the kind of care they need and receive, and can be grouped accordingly, residents in aged care facilities have largely common areas of dependency in which their degrees of dependency differ, so that their care needs in each area can be rated on a continuous or ordinal scale and summed across all areas. The additive model was also found to explain slightly more of the variance in the cost/time variable. It was also considered that it would be easier in practice for staff and providers to "evolve" from the existing scales to the single new Resident Classification Scale (RCS). The familiar four level ratings were retained for most items.

When the "mathematical" part of the classification development was completed, the federal Department of Health and Aged Care decided that it would be appropriate to split the continuous distribution of scores into eight care categories and payment bands. The cut-off points for these bands and the subsequent level of payment for each category were set with a view to minimizing changes in funding received by facilities under the old and new systems, and a need for fiscal responsibility. Collapsing the previous five RCI categories and the four PCAI categories into eight categories, with similar upper and lower funding limits, also appeared to address the overlap between the lowest RCI category and the highest PCAI category.

The RCS was phased in from October 1997. All newly admitted residents were classified using the RCS, and all existing residents were reclassified at the time of their annual reviews, unless a marked change in care need warranted earlier reviews. Given the difficulties encountered when developing any new classification system, the experience with the RCS has been judged as reasonably successful in so far as it has produced a redistribution of funding within the residential care system in the desired direction. Residents at the lower level of the nursing home scale (RCI) tended to receive less funding than previously because they could now rate as low as RCS 7, compared to the lowest level in the dual-funding system of RCI 5. Conversely, more dependent residents in hostels moved up the new scale, and the proportion of hostel residents assessed at RCS 3 received an immediate and significant increase in funding. Taken over the entire residential care system, funding increased in the first year of the RCI by approximately $70m on a base of $2,874m in 1997-98 (Cuthbertson, Lindsay-Smith, & Rosewarne, 1998).

The RCS was generally well accepted by residential care providers, but a number of issues identified in the course of implementation lead to a review. The author was a member of the review team that presented its report in mid 1998 (Cuthbertson, Lindsay-Smith, & Rosewarne, 1998). The scope of the review was limited to essentially technical aspects of the RCS, and only minor changes resulted, involving the combination of some items, changes in some item ratings, and revision of guidelines to give greater clarity for use of the RCS. Table 1 presents a summary of the final items in the RCS, the ratings, and the regression weights.

Classification Processes

The resident classification process involves a number of steps, and there is provision for monitoring of classification at the level of the individual resident, the facility, and the system overall. The first step, mandatory assessment by an ACAT, has been noted above.

The second step occurs after admission when facility staff completes the RCS. The appraisal of the resident's dependency and care needs extends over the first month after admission. A detailed manual sets out a guide for rating of residents on the 20 RCS items that cover comprehension, communication, continence, behavior, activities of daily living, therapy, technical nursing requirements, medication, and social and human needs. These ratings translate into a weighted score on each item (see Table 1), and the item scores are summed and the total score determines the classification into one of eight categories and the associated level of funding.

Although there is now no longer a tie between the facility in which care is provided and resident care categories, the vast majority of nursing home residents rate in categories one to four. Most hostel residents are in categories five to eight, but an increasing proportion are in categories three and four as aging

TABLE 1. Resident Classification Scale Items and Weightings

RCS Items	Weightings			
	A	B	C	D
	usually independent	requires some assistance	requires major assistance	requires extensive assistance
1. Communication	0	0.28	0.36	0.83
2. Mobility	0	1.19	1.54	1.82
3. Meals and drinks	0	0.67	0.75	2.65
4. Personal hygiene	0	**5.34**	**14.17**	14.61
5. Toileting	0	**5.98**	**10.65**	13.70
6. Bladder management	0	2.22	3.81	4.20
7. Bowel management	0	**3.32**	**5.72**	6.30
8. Understanding & undertaking living activities	0	0.79	1.11	3.40
9. Problem wandering or intrusive behavior	0	0.80	1.58	4.00
10. Verbally disruptive or noisy	0	1.19	1.76	4.60
11. Physically aggressive	0	2.34	2.69	3.05
12. Emotional dependence	0	0.28	1.50	3.84
13. Danger to self or others	0	1.11	1.54	1.98
14. Other behavior	0	0.91	1.82	2.61
15. Social and human needs–care recipient	0	0.95	1.98	3.01
16. Social and human needs–families & friends	0	0.28	0.55	0.91
17. Medication	0	**0.79**	**8.55**	11.40
18. Technical and complex nursing procedures	0	**1.54**	**5.54**	11.16
19. Therapy	0	3.64	6.10	7.01
20. Other services	0	0.71	1.46	2.93
Total	0	34.33	73.18	104.00

in place proceeds. Once established, the classification remains valid for one year unless there is a significant change in care needs. Review by an ACAT is required if a subsequent RCS appraisal of a resident admitted to a low-care facility results in rating for high-level care, either in the same facility or through transfer to a high-care facility.

Classification Review

RCS categories are reviewed at two levels. First, the distribution of RCS categories across all facilities is monitored. As well as watching for "classification creep," which can result in substantial increases in outlays, this monitoring can identify facilities in which RCS profiles differ from other similar facilities. This monitoring provides the basis of a risk management strategy for targeting facilities for RCS reviews because there are only approximately 50 review officers to cover nearly 140,000 RCS claims annually. Reports from the quality assurance process also inform the risk management strategy and provide one of the few links between the resident classification and quality assurance processes.

Once in a facility, the review officers check only a sample of RCS ratings and scores. The review officers are employees of the federal Department of Health and Aged Care, and most have qualifications in aged care nursing. The review of individual RCS forms and associated documentation is intended as an audit or validation of the documentation on which the facility bases its RCS classification claim. Validation is thus concerned with system performance as much as with checking on individual resident ratings. The review process is well established and has worked reasonably well on the basis of professionalism of nursing staff, the skills of the review officers, and open communication between staff and review officers. There are nonetheless a number of ongoing concerns to providers and to the government as the source of funds.

First, review officers are reliant on care staff for the care plan documentation on which they base their validation, and residents are not assessed directly. For example, a facility may assess that a person needs to be transferred with the use of lifting equipment. Even if a review officer observes the resident concerned transferring independently, the legislative reliance on written material makes it difficult to question the RCS score if it is well documented. This difficulty is also complicated by the fact that the review officer's visit is likely to be some time after the date the assessment was made by the facility.

A second problem area is that documentation can be developed "creatively," and it is difficult to ascertain if residents are in fact receiving the level of care as detailed in the care plan. The current system is based on documented interventions, so to increase funding for a resident, a facility need only develop, for example, a therapy program to claim that therapy services are being provided to residents. If the program is based on an assessment, includes appropriate aims, and is supervised by an appropriately qualified person, a claim is allowed. While this example could be seen as a positive as it provides an incentive for facilities to consider the provision of additional care to residents, it creates a number of problems because there is no quality control on the program that is provided, there is nothing to ensure the assessment is valid, and often no assurance that the program is in fact delivered as frequently as the plan specifies.

A third problem is that, although the RCS appraisal by staff was intended to flow directly from the documentation used to assess care needs, the RCS documentation process has moved away from the collection of information to develop care plans to guide clinical and social supports for individuals towards a model of collection of information to support funding claims. Some facilities then develop two sets of documentation–one for the funding claim preparation and the other for staff providing the direct care.

There are also limitations in the review process. Although review officers have wide experience, their review of documentation is to some extent subjective in nature, and with over 50 staff involved nationally, it is difficult to maintain a consistent and reliable approach to the reviews. Rather than the review process being a thorough check on care planning and service delivery, the main disincentive to over claiming is that if the review results in a downgrading to a lower care category, the facility retroactively loses the funding that has been received since the claim was made.

RCS documentation review is the only method currently used to validate the distribution of recurrent expenditure on residential care, estimated at $3.5 billion in 1999-2000. RCS review is even more important in the integrated residential care system than in the previous dual-funding system in which the number of residents for whom higher levels of funding could be claimed was tied to the number of nursing home places. The first year of integration of nursing homes and hostels into a single system saw a substantial increase in recurrent funding due to the reclassification of former hostel residents to higher levels of care, but subsequent experiences suggest that this was largely a one-off adjustment. However, without external controls to prevent the documentation of rising care needs, systematic increases in RCS claims have the potential significantly to increase government expenditure since there is no cap on the outlays resulting from higher classifications.

QUALITY ASSURANCE

History

The present quality assurance process involves the participation of providers in a system that has evolved over the last 15 years. Prior to 1987, rudimentary quality assurance in nursing homes and hostels was undertaken by state government authorities responsible for hospitals and other health care facilities, and whose regulatory functions focused on care inputs and compliance with state regulations, mainly relating to physical facility standards.

In 1987, the federal government initiated a quality assurance system that specified a set of Outcome Standards that were audited by Standards Monitoring Teams. These teams comprised government officials, at least one of whom was a registered nurse. The standard monitoring process realized considerable gains in quality of care, and evaluations reported positive outcomes in establishing an effective regulatory dialogue between providers and regulators (Braithwaite, Braithwaite, Gibson, & Makkai, 1994; Braithwaite, 1998).

In 1996, following the change of federal government, the standards monitoring process was extended to a more comprehensive system that provided for both *certification* of physical facilities and *accreditation* of care standards. The new system required all facilities to meet both certification and accreditation standards as a condition for continued receipt of federal funding from January 1, 2001. While in the United States "certification" is used to designate approval of facilities for public funding and "accreditation" refers to voluntary participation in independent standards compliance activities, the terms have somewhat different meanings in the Australian quality assurance system because both certification and accreditation are mandatory.

The Accreditation Process

The Aged Care Standards and Accreditation Agency was established by the federal government to drive the provision of quality aged care services at the same time as removing government from the role of direct regulator. The Agency is charged with developing and maintaining a quality accreditation program for all residential aged care facilities. Quality assessors are employed by the Agency, and they visit facilities to conduct assessments. This mainly involves a review of documentation, including random selection care plans. The assessment also involves discussions with staff, residents, and family members to ascertain if the care as outlined in the documentation is being delivered and how quality standards are being met and maintained. As with the previous standards monitoring system, the new program has built-in incentives and educational elements, as well as penalties for non-compliance.

Full accreditation is achieved if facilities meet the standards for certification of buildings and accreditation of care standards in the four domains of:

1. Management systems, staffing, and organizational development
2. Health and personal care of residents
3. Resident lifestyle
4. Physical environment and safe systems

Within these areas, there are 44 standards, and a number of outcomes are expected to be achieved within each standard. Full details of the standards and related documentation are available via the Internet sites for the Standards and Accreditation Agency (http://www.accreditation.aust.com) and the federal Department of Health and Aged Care (http://www.health.gov.au/acc/manuals/sgr/sgrindex.htm).

The assessment process involves several steps. Each facility seeking accreditation first completes a fully documented self-assessment on the standards and the outcomes it expects to achieve. This self-assessment is then compared to the ratings provided by an independent assessor who visits the facility. Facilities must also show that they are participating in continuous improvement activities. The independent assessor gives a rating on each expected outcome within each standard and a summary rating in each of the four domains. Finally, each facility receives an overall accreditation rating on all domains at the level of commendable, satisfactory, unacceptable, or critical. A commendable or satisfactory overall rating gives accreditation for three years. If ratings are below satisfactory in some standards, accreditation is granted for one year only, and regular monitoring is conducted. One or more ratings at the critical level means a facility has failed accreditation.

The accreditation system is designed to raise the quality of resident care throughout the aged care sector and uses both a carrot and a stick to this end. The carrot comes by way of motivating providers and staff to achieve an overall rating of commendable and thereby place their facility in the top 10% of all facilities. The stick comes from having to undergo a further full accreditation if a provisional accreditation is given for only one year, or worse, from the risk of losing funding if accreditation is failed.

The outcome of accreditation surveys conducted to the end of December 2000, to meet the deadline of January 1, 2001 for continued funding, indicates that most facilities were able to achieve the required standards. Only 10% of homes achieved a commendable rating on at least one of the four standards domains, and fully 88% achieved satisfactory ratings. Some 4% of facilities were rated as unacceptable on any one domain, and so received only one year's accreditation. Only 2% were rated as critical; of these, several were granted an "exceptional circumstances" determination on grounds such as not being able to complete building works, and were allowed to continue to operate on the condition that the shortcomings in the physical environment and safety systems were remedied within six months.

The eventual outcomes for the remaining facilities that either failed to meet the accreditation standards or did not even seek accreditation are unclear. Such facilities will no longer receive federal funding, unless they are covered by an exceptional circumstances determination. No official figures are kept on the facilities that fail accreditation, so while the process of exit from the formal residential care system has achieved the federal government's goals of improving quality of care, it is not known whether unaccredited facilities have closed or have continued as unfunded services operating as supported residential services at the bottom end of the market.

The new system has been effective in withdrawing federal funding from poor quality homes that anticipated they would be unable to meet the standards, or that sought accreditation but failed. It has also recognized the best homes. However, among the very large group of homes in the middle, there is a wide range from those that almost reached commendable standards to those that only reached satisfactory, and this lack of differentiation has been a point of criticism in the industry. All the satisfactory homes gained three years accreditation, and it remains to be seen how far the accreditation system will realize its goals for continuous quality improvement over the next few years.

FUTURE PROSPECTS AND POSSIBLE DEVELOPMENTS

The Assessment Instrument

After a period of considerable change from late 1997, the resident classification and quality assurance systems that are now in place seem set to remain stable for the foreseeable future. While a report on the restructuring of residential care over the last two years has been recently released, it is unlikely that further major changes will be made. Adjustments made in the course of implementation have addressed many concerns, and by the beginning of 2001, both systems were seen to be operating relatively smoothly. Although the prospects for change appear limited in the short term, there are several areas that require attention if the current systems are to be effective and sustainable over the longer term.

There are three aspects of the RCS that remain problematic and that could be addressed directly. First, the RCS displays an internal inconsistency regarding its purpose. While the RCS is supposed to be an instrument that assesses care needs directly related to the cost of care, it also has a number of items designed to encourage best practice in the provision of the care. For example, many questions provide a greater score for staff efforts designed to encourage and support a resident to provide his or her own care. While this is a better outcome in a care quality sense (compared with staff completing the function for the resident), it is problematic that the RCS is used in this manner.

Second, the number of items in the RCS (20) is unnecessarily large. A reduced scale could achieve the same classification result and remove a considerable part of the extensive documentation required for validation, a source of much complaint from nursing staff. Many items were included in the RCS largely for face validity but are either highly correlated or make a very small contribution to the overall cost of care. A modified 7-item version of the RCS developed by the author resulted in little loss of information, a much greater focus on the assessment of resident dependency and care needs, and elimination of items covering care services to be delivered by staff.

The third problem with the structure of the RCS is that it presents two incentives for gaming. Table 1 shows there are substantial differences between weightings for the rating levels on some items (shown in bold). These differences create an incentive for providers to maximize ratings on items for which a C rather than a B rating has a large impact on the RCS score and hence on funding. The increments among the eight bands of funding are also uneven, compounding the incentive to game the system in a way that would not be so compelling with evenly graduated, and possibly a larger number of, categories with incremental funding increases.

The Assessment Process

A further set of developments involving collection and transfer of information among the processes of ACAT assessment, resident classification, and quality assurance could address some of the remaining problems in these processes. As the horizontal arrows in Figure 1 show, these developments could bring the three currently separate processes together to promote quality of care.

Client dependency data collected in the ACAT assessment provide two options for a reference point that could be used in resident classification. The first option would see the ACAT assessment used to determine the RCS category and funding level of the resident with a "review if required" option for facilities. Facilities would have the option of submitting a "review" if they felt the ACAT assessment and subsequent funding level did not adequately measure residents' care needs. Resident funding would stay the same after the ACAT assessment unless facilities submitted this "review" request, eliminating the need for facilities to prepare documentation for funding purposes except for residents for whom a review was requested. The usual documentation for care plans would still be required as a part of professional standards of care. While this approach would add to the role of the ACATs, linking RCS appraisal to the ACAT assessment could remove the need for facility visits by review officers other than in exceptional cases where an ACAT and facility assessment are irreconcilable. Compared to the current system, this approach could achieve more consistency in funding for the same resident profile, no matter where the resident was located, with variations in cost better explained by resident characteristics than by provider-related factors.

The second option would involve linking the ACAT Minimum Data Set on assessments to the RCS assessment conducted by facilities, via an administrative system. The data matching could be limited to five to seven key items and so be much more economical regarding time and effort than the present system. Facilities would still be required to use an RCS-style instrument on all residents, but reviews by review officers would be required only when the facility-based RCS assessment was significantly higher than the ACAT assessment. As in the first option, the need for reviews would be significantly reduced.

The second area for further development concerns the issue about whether funding on the basis of dependency creates dependency. Rather than being resolved, this issue has been confounded by some of the RCS items framed with reference to care provided rather than the dependency of the resident, with the intention of rewarding facilities that provided care to maintain and promote independence in functioning. In practice, this approach has created problems because it is harder to audit whether or not care is actually provided via a documentation review; the documentation is provided by care staff and is open to a degree of manipulation. A more dependency-focused RCS could conceivably provide the kind of information that would enable the funding system and the quality assurance process to reward facilities that achieved positive resident outcomes and promoted independence.

A final gap is that while the current system of funding is based on assessment of the individual resident's needs, the quality assurance process is based on an assessment of the quality of the care and infrastructure provided by a facility as a whole, and there is no link between the individual-based and facility-wide systems. A less well-managed, poorly equipped facility receives the same funding for a RCS category 1 resident as a well-managed, extensively equipped facility, even though the standards system may rate the two facilities differently. While it would be unfair to residents with the same care needs if the lower quality facility received less funding than a high-quality-of-care facility, the present situation may provide a perverse incentive for skimping, that is, providing the minimum level of service and care quality to a resident. A quality-based funding approach would need to add a "bonus" framework as an additional component to the RCS funding model. In such an approach, the standards monitoring and accreditation assessment process would be the means of linking outputs and outcomes in terms of quality of care services to the inputs of care, with reference back to resident classification as a funding allocation mechanism. This approach could capture the effects of use of physiotherapists, skilled nursing staff, documentation of care practices and so on, on quality of care. For the time being, however, classification remains largely separate from accreditation because there is no formal connection between these processes.

Finally, it is essential to develop clinical indicators related directly to the care standards covered in the accreditation process if quality of care is to improve further. The provision of general training programs and improving knowledge does not necessarily lead to improvements in care practices and care outcomes. Apart from the necessary changes to overall management, care models, and practices, it is essential to have measures of the relationships among care inputs, outputs, and outcomes of the care that is delivered. Without some systematic measurement of the current status of care programs, it is difficult to know what outcomes are achieved and whether or not quality of care is improving. To this end, it will be necessary to develop benchmarking methods for measuring critical aspects of quality of care and to assess performance against these standards. This measurement approach could be used to help service providers focus on continuous quality improvement by examining where they are now, individually and collectively, across the whole aged care system, and identifying what needs to be done to improve their performance.

REFERENCES

Australian Institute of Health and Welfare (AIHW) (1997). *Nursing Homes in Australia, 1995-96: Aged Care Statistics Series No. 1.* Canberra: AIHW and Department of Health and Family Services.

Australian Institute of Health and Welfare (AIHW) (1998a). *Nursing Homes in Australia, 1996-97: A Statistical Overview.* AIHW Cat. No. AGE 9.

Australian Institute of Health and Welfare (AIHW) (1998b). *Hostels in Australia, 1996-97: A Statistical Overview.* AIHW Cat. No. AGE 10.

Australian Institute of Health and Welfare (AIHW) (1999). *Residential Care in Australia, 1998-99: A Statistical Overview.* AIHW Cat. No. AGE 16.

Australian Institute of Health and Welfare (AIHW) (2001). *Australia's Welfare 2001: Services and Assistance.* Canberra: AIHW.

Braithwaite, V., Braithwaite, J., Gibson, D., & Makkai, T. (1994). Regulatory styles, motivational postures and nursing home compliance. *Law and Policy, 16*: 363-94.

Braithwaite, J. (1998). Regulation and quality in aged care: A cross national perspective. *Australasian Journal on Ageing, 17*(4): 172-176.

Cuthbertson S., Lindsay-Smith E., & Rosewarne, R. C. (1998). Review of the Resident Classification Scale. *Aged and Community Care Service Development and Evaluation Reports*, No. 36. Canberra: AusInfo.

Hindle, D. (1996). *Analysis of Different Ways of Developing a Single Instrument for Classification of Nursing Home and Hostel Residents.* Canberra: Commonwealth Department of Health and Family Services.

Rhys Hearn, C. (1997). *Development of a Single Instrument for the Classification of Nursing Home and Hostel Residents.* Perth: Aged Care Research and Evaluation Unit, University of Western Australia.

Long-Term Care Policy for Elders in Hong Kong

Iris Chi, DSW

Director, Centre on Aging,
University of Hong Kong

SUMMARY. The context in which aged care policy is being developed in Hong Kong is characterized not only by rapid demographic aging and social change, but also by new political and administrative systems being built on a colonial legacy. This article begins with a description of the demographic profile and trends in population aging, noting particular dif-

---

Professor Iris Chi received her Bachelor of Social Science at the Chinese University of Hong Kong in 1978 and obtained her Doctorate in Social Welfare from the University of California, Los Angeles, in 1985. Since 1998, she has been Professor and Director of the Centre on Ageing at the University of Hong Kong. She has published over 50 articles in regional and international refereed journals; other publications include 14 edited books and monographs and 12 book chapters. She has been an invited keynote speaker at many international and regional conferences and has been appointed to policy and academic consultant positions, including membership in the Elderly Commission of the Hong Kong Special Administrative Region, special advisor on aging to the WHO and the UN, advisory board member of the National U. S. Academy of Certified Care Managers, associate fellow of interRAI, and advisor to the International Association of Gerontology Asia-Oceania Region. She is a member of the editorial board of international journals, and has held positions as an honorary professor and research fellow of international research centers on aging, including the University of Victoria, BC, Canada.

Professor Chi can be contacted at the Department of Social Work and Social Administration, The University of Hong Kong, Pokfulam Rd., Hong Kong (E-mail: irischi@hku.hk).

[Haworth co-indexing entry note]: "Long-Term Care Policy for Elders in Hong Kong." Chi, Iris. Co-published simultaneously in *Journal of Aging & Social Policy* (The Haworth Press, Inc.) Vol. 13, No. 2/3, 2001, pp. 137-153; and: *Long-Term Care in the 21st Century: Perspectives from Around the Asia-Pacific Rim* (ed: Iris Chi, Kalyani K. Mehta, and Anna L. Howe) The Haworth Press, Inc., 2001, pp. 137-153. Single or multiple copies of this article are available for a fee from The Haworth Document Delivery Service [1-800-HAWORTH, 9:00 a.m. - 5:00 p.m. (EST). E-mail address: getinfo@haworthpressinc.com].

137

ferences in marriage and family formation that differentiate Hong Kong from other developed countries and that also show marked changes between generations. While past social policies can be credited with contributing to the achievement of high life expectancy in Hong Kong, these policies were unevenly developed, with little provision for income security in old age or for long-term care. Both issues have come to the fore in policy development in recent years, culminating in the formation of the Elderly Commission in 1997 and revitalizing the level of attention given to developing community care. A clear policy agenda has been drawn up to promote the development of a long-term care system, addressing issues of integration; role differentiation for assessment and service provision, including new contractual arrangements; quality assurance; and financing. The political and administrative changes are seen to present opportunities for containing residential care and forging a care system founded on community services. *[Article copies available for a fee from The Haworth Document Delivery Service: 1-800-HAWORTH. E-mail address: <getinfo@haworthpressinc.com> Website: <http://www.HaworthPress.com> © 2001 by The Haworth Press, Inc. All rights reserved.]*

KEYWORDS. Community care, contracting, Elderly Commission, family care, public funding

THE POLICY CONTEXT

The context in which aged care policy is being developed in Hong Kong is characterized not only by rapid demographic aging and social change associated with continuing economic development, but by new political and administrative systems being built on a colonial legacy. The former changes mean that purposeful attention must be given to the role of the family in care of the elderly, while the latter changes present opportunities for containing the as-yet relatively-limited provision of residential care and forging a care system that is founded on community services.

Demographic Profile and Trends

Hong Kong has experienced a steady and significant growth in its elderly population. The percentage of persons aged 65 and above has increased from 8.8% of the population in 1991 to 10% in 1996 and is expected to rise to 11.2% in 2006 and 13.3% in 2016 (Census and Statistics Department, 1998). Traditionally, old age in Hong Kong is defined as 60 years or older. In 1998, 15% of the population was elderly (Census and Statistics Department, 1998). Between 1986 and 1996, the population aged 60 or over grew by 39%. By 2006, it is estimated that there will be 1,093,200 people aged 60 and above in Hong Kong, a further increase of 23% over the 1996 figure. Table 1 shows the population aging in Hong Kong between the years 1996 to 2016.

Health Status and Social Profile

Hong Kong's population enjoys one of the longest life expectancies in the world. As of 1999, female life expectancy at birth was 82.3 years and 76.9 years for males, and it is projected that by 2016, life expectancy for females will be 83.4 and 78.1 for males (Hong Kong Population Projections, 1997-2016).

Based on these figures, Hong Kong will be facing an increasingly large population of elderly people. The average annual growth rate of the population aged 60 and above is estimated to be 2.5% from 1996 to 2001 and 1.8% from 2001 to 2006. The 75-and-above age group shows greater annual growth, averaging 5.2% and 4.6% for the two time periods, respectively. This trend will likely continue for the next 20 years, resulting in aging of the aged population. This outcome is of considerable significance for policy and service planning because it is the very old who make the heaviest demands on health and social services (Chi & Chui, 1999).

In terms of gender distribution, in 1996 men accounted for 47% of the elderly population and women 53%. The gender ratio is much more evenly balanced than in western aging countries, due in large part to the large-scale immigration of male laborers to Hong Kong from China over the post-war years. In 2006, these gender balances will be 49% men and 51% women, evidencing the continuing increase in the number of elderly men ahead of elderly women. Contrary to expectations in line with western patterns that the population would become more pronouncedly female as it ages, the figures in Hong Kong suggest this even gender balance will be maintained. This may partially be due to the aged population still being relatively young, so that gender differences that show up most clearly over age 80 are not yet evident (Chi & Chui, 1999).

Marital status patterns also differ from western countries. The proportion of elderly people who are widowed has declined from 33% in 1981 to 28% in 1996, and on the other hand, the proportion currently married has increased from 61% to 66% in 1996. The proportion never married has been consistently low for the past 15 years, at between 4% and 5% of the elderly population. Analysis of the proportions never married by gender for the years 1986 and 1996 shows that single marital status among women decreased from 6.5% to

TABLE 1. Population Aging in Hong Kong, 1996-2016

Year	1996		2006		2016	
Population aged	'000	%	'000	%	'000	%
60-64	300	4.0	300	3.6	500	6.4
65-69	200	3.6	200	3.2	400	5.0
70 and above	400	6.5	600	8.0	700	8.3
Total aged 60+	900	14.1	1,100	14.8	1,600	19.7

3%, whereas for men it increased from 4% to 5%. These figures suggest that more older people in Hong Kong will be moving into old age as partners in married couples than in the west (Chi & Chui, 1999).

THE LEGACY OF PAST SOCIAL POLICIES

The social profile of the current generation of elderly in Hong Kong reflects the uneven development of social policies covering housing, education, employment, and access to pensions in the past. The majority of elderly people are adequately housed, but since no pension system was in place until 2000, there are many low-income elderly relying on social assistance. The pace of economic and social development over the last 20 years or more has left many of the elderly behind, resulting in major intergenerational differences in education levels and standards of living.

Housing

The Hong Kong government historically has had an extensive public housing program for its citizens for many years. Approximately half of the elderly population is currently living in government rented or subsidized flats, and only one third of the elderly people own their homes (Chi & Chow, 1997). Access to adequate housing on the part of older and younger generations has contributed to significant changes in the living arrangements of elderly people in Hong Kong in the past two decades, and the traditional extended family is no longer the norm in family living arrangements.

Living Arrangements

The proportion of all households that were nuclear families had already reached just on 60% by 1986, so the margin for further change is more limited, with 63% being nuclear families in 1996. There are significant age and gender differences in living arrangements among the older population. More elderly people are living alone or with spouse only, with a total of 270,000 now in these living arrangements. As in 1997, some 10% of those aged 65 and older lived alone, and about 15% lived with their spouses only (Census and Statistics Department, 1998). Among those who live with others, including those living with adult children, many are actually living with another elderly person such as a sibling, and among the very elderly, adult children can also be aged over 65. The older group, aged 80 and above, tends to live alone, and the females also tend to live alone (Chi & Chow, 1997).

Education

A high proportion of the elderly population has never received schooling or formal education in Hong Kong. In 1995, this group constituted 45% of the elderly population. While the proportion of elderly who has attained primary school education is increasing, the proportion with secondary and tertiary education has remained relatively constant since 1990. While it is anticipated that the proportion who has had no education will continue to decrease and the proportion with primary education will increase, the proportion with secondary or tertiary education is likely to remain constant for the next 10 years (Chi & Chui, 1999).

Employment

Elderly people account for only some 5% of Hong Kong's wage-earning employed population since 1990. Of those employed elderly persons, the majority earn between US$500 to US$780 a month. There is a slow but steady trend towards higher earnings of more than US$780 to US$1950 a month, possibly due to better job opportunities resulting from the higher educational attainment of the 60 to 64 age group. Although monthly employment earnings have increased, the labor participation rate of people age 65 and above decreased from 19.5% in 1986 to 9.8% in 1996 and decreased further to 5.5% in 1999. The decrease in the labor force participation rate is found in both genders (Chi & Chui, 1999).

Social Security

In contrast to the extensive government involvement in housing, Hong Kong had no mandatory retirement pension scheme until 2000; hence, most elderly people are not financially independent. The majority are supported by their families, and very few are able to live on their own savings. As a consequence, elderly persons in Hong Kong have become the poorest segment in the society. The social security scheme in Hong Kong takes the form of public assistance, and it is the only safety net for poor people. The scheme is mainly funded by taxation, and it provides a minimal level of support through a means test. As in the year 1999, 18% of the elderly population aged 65 and above were recipients of the Comprehensive Social Security Allowance (CSSA) (Social Welfare Department, 1999). These 132,800 individuals constitute more than 65% of the total public assistance cases. It is anticipated that elderly persons will continue to be the major recipients of the public assistance for the coming years, not only causing a significant burden to the government but also affecting the quality of life of these older people.

Health Care

Hong Kong's medical and health system is unusual in that it is mainly publicly funded. This situation can be attributed largely to the British colonial administration under which the basic health care system was established. Private practitioners provide most of the primary health care, and less than 15% is provided by the Department of Health. Elderly people are the main consumers of the public primary health care system, and they pay one third of the cost of treatment and medicines; the remainder of the cost is covered by public funds. The secondary and tertiary medical care, on the other hand, is provided mainly by the Hospital Authority, and the private sector plays a very insignificant role. A similar funding arrangement applies to the Hospital Authority's health care services, which are heavily subsidized with public funds. Less than 20% of Hong Kong's citizens have any type of medical and health insurance, mostly through private insurance programs (Harvard Report, 1999). No scheme is available in Hong Kong at the moment to provide long-term care insurance coverage.

CURRENT POLICY COMMITMENTS

Administrative Developments

Commitment to aged care on the part of the Hong Kong government has not been very high in the past, but this has changed markedly in recent years, and there have been a number of significant institutional developments including policy statements, the establishment of a mandatory provident fund, and an Elderly Commission.

The annual policy addresses by the Chief Executive in 1997, 1998, and 1999 all included statements identifying "caring for the elderly" as one of the strategic policy objectives. This period spans the transfer from the British Colonial government to the Chinese Special Administrative Region (SAR) Government. In 1999, the SAR government pledged to provide the elderly with a sense of security, a sense of belonging, and a feeling of happiness and worthiness (Policy Address, 1999).

A mandatory provident fund (MPF) scheme, which is a compulsory private saving plan, began at the end of year 2000. Although this is a very modest private saving scheme, it is hoped that in 15 years, Hong Kong will accumulate enough funds to provide a minimum retirement protection for its senior citizens.

A high-level advisory body, the Elderly Commission, was set up in July 1997 with the following mission:

- To formulate a comprehensive policy;
- To coordinate the planning and development of services;
- To recommend priorities; and
- To monitor the implementation of policies and programs.

While the Elderly Commission spans all spheres of government, providers' sectors, and community representation, the Health and Welfare Bureau has the major responsibility in setting aged care policies for Hong Kong. There are three major executive departments under the Bureau: the Department of Health, the Department of Social Welfare, and the Hospital Authority.

Policy Objectives

The objective of elderly services in Hong Kong is to promote well-being of the elderly through care in the community and by the community (Hong Kong Government, 1997). Community care has been the policy for elderly services since the 1970s. The cardinal principle of community care is to facilitate the elderly and their family caregivers to take care of them in the home environment and to provide residential care when family and community support services cannot meet the need (Social Welfare Department, 1999). While this policy objective has only been put into effect on a limited scale to date, the way is open to build a system that is strongly oriented to community care. Realizing this outcome will depend on both the policy decisions taken and the funding arrangements put in place.

FINANCING

Financing arrangements for long-term care are more varied than for health care services and are interrelated with the structure of the delivery system.

Long-term care programs are delivered through a variety of providers, including the Hospital Authority, Department of Health, Social Welfare Department, non-governmental organizations, private sector operators and volunteers, neighborhood support groups, and family caregivers. Public funding is provided for both residential care services and community support services, with different financing arrangements for providers in the public, "subvented" or not-for-profit sector, and for providers in the private for-profit sector. In 1996, total expenditure reached US$251.7m, of which 64% went to residential care and 36% to community care.

Community Care

The division of community care between community health programs and community support services is paralleled by a division of providers. Community health programs for elderly people are provided by hospitals and the Department of Health, and include Community Geriatric Assessment Teams, community nursing services, home-based rehabilitation, elderly health centers, and elderly health outreach teams. Community support services, on the other hand, are mainly provided by non-government organizations that receive most of their funding from the government.

The range of community support services and the allocation of funding between them are set out in Table 2. Expansion of services is dependent on government funding, and commitments to 2002/03 are focused on expansion of more intensive care services and away from social centers, with planned additional provision for five multi-service centers, seven-day centers, and four home-care teams.

The Hong Kong Government re-engineered the home help service in 1999 by separating the two main components, namely meals services and home-care services through competitive bidding. Altogether, 25 home-care teams were set up since December 1999, and another 25 meal teams started in early 2000. This initiative aimed to add value through the provision of between 5% to 12.5% additional service units at no extra cost. It also saw extension of service hours to cover the evening, more systematic training plans, and stronger collaboration with local medical and paramedical personnel. Instead of setting rigid professional staffing provisions, the new funding arrangements allow the operating agencies to decide on how they deploy their human resources.

Residential Care

As detailed in Table 3, there are four bands of residential care services and these apply across the private, subvented or not-for-profit, and public sectors. The subvented sector receives operating subsidies related to the physical struc-

TABLE 2. Provision and Funding of Community Support Services, January 2000

Type of service	Provision	Professional staffing provision	Expenditure	
			US$m	%
Social Center for the Elderly	211 centers	211	22.0	24.1
Multi-service Center	32 centers	192	17.0	18.6
Day Care	31 centers	86	12.2	13.4
Home-help Team	138 teams	138	)	
Home-care Team	25 teams	Subject to proposals of operating agencies	) 40.0)	43.9
Total			91.2	100.0

ture of facilities, especially the amount of space available per resident, and to staffing ratios, but these are essentially historic and not systematically related to either the level of care provided or quality of care. Public funding is also provided to some private sector homes through a "bought places" scheme, with funding along the same lines.

Private homes for the aged cater to some 22,800 individuals and provide 55% of all residential care places, across the full spectrum of levels of care. Although privately run as profit-making enterprises, about one third of places are in homes that meet quality requirements (see below) for direct subsidy through the "bought place scheme." Another third of places are in homes of lower quality and do not qualify for this scheme, but they are nonetheless subsidized indirectly through CSSA, which provides income support to residents and which is used to pay the fees charged by providers. The remaining third of homes are fully self-financing, and cater to elderly people from upper- and middle-class families, with fees paid either by the elderly or by their adult children.

Subvented facilities provide three levels of care. At all levels, the subsidies from government mean that residents have to pay only basic costs of living, and places in subvented homes are sought on these grounds as well as for the higher levels of care made possible through the subsidies.

- *Hostels and homes for the aged* provide the lowest level of care; they account for 12% of all places and receive close to 15% of the public funds that go to the subvented sector.

- *Care and attention homes and homes combining care and attention and nursing care* account for 30% of places and absorb about 70% of the public funding that goes to the subvented sector.
- *Nursing homes* account for just over 3% of places and are even more costly per bed, and so absorb 14% of public funding in the subvented sector.

The provision of more care services increases the cost and adds to the quality of care in subvented facilities at all levels of care; they are less costly for residents since the operating subsidies mean that residents have to meet only basic living costs. In care and attention homes, for example, fees paid by residents account for only about 10% of the total cost.

Infirmary beds are provided by some of the public hospitals in Hong Kong and were considered as part of residential care services in the past. However, the function of these hospital services has recently been redefined as serving only those who are capable of active rehabilitation, and so length of stay will be reduced.

Quality of Care

Quality of care in private homes is closely related to funding and ranges from good in self-financing homes that charge very high fees, through satisfac-

TABLE 3. Provision and Funding of Residential Care Services, January 2000

Type of home	No. of facilities	No. of beds	% of beds	Expenditure US$m	%	Av. cost per place to govt. $
Private						
Bought places	n.a	~ 7,600	~18	n.a.	n.a.	n.a.
Mainly CSSA	n.a	~ 7,600	~18	nil	nil	nil
Self financing	n.a	~ 7,600	~18	nil	nil	nil
Total	450	22,800	55			
Subvented						
Hostels	21	3,029	7	12.9	8.0	4,259
Homes for the Aged	17	1,983	5	10.5	6.5	5,295
Combined homes	40	5,779	14	49.7	30.9	8,600
Care-and-attention	41	6,195	15	65.5	40.8	10,573
Nursing Homes	6	1,400	3	21.9	13.6	16,000
Total	125	18,386	45	160.5	100.0	
Total	575	41,186	100			

tory in the "bought place" homes, to very basic in those that cater mainly to CSSA residents.

The substandard private homes that charge relatively low fees tend to provide poor quality of care but have been growing rapidly. The poor quality of care in these private homes has made the headlines on several occasions, and on April 1, 1995, the government introduced the Residential Care Homes (Elderly Persons) Ordinance.

This Ordinance regulates the operation of homes by license or provides a certificate of exemption (CoE) for a specified period. The Ordinance covers only the physical aspects of the home safety such as to ensure building and fire safety, space standard, and staffing ratio. Most of the private homes could not obtain a license to operate and had to apply for exemptions. Legally speaking, these homes cannot operate if they do not meet the standards set by the Social Welfare Department. In reality, none of these homes has been closed down due to the poor standard or poor quality of care. Instead, a one-off Financial Assistance Scheme was introduced in June 1995 to help private homes to reach the standards (Social Welfare Department, 1997). By December 31, 1999, 431 homes were licensed, and of these, 230 had been granted CoEs. The government was determined to assist all homes to get their licenses in early 2001 (Hong Kong Government, 1999).

CHALLENGES FACED BY HONG KONG

The six challenges to caring for the elderly faced by Hong Kong are summarized as:

1. Rapid aging of the aged population and increasing life expectancy;
2. Low social economic status and financial capability among the aged;
3. Increasing number of elderly with chronic diseases and functional disabilities;
4. Weakening family support;
5. No infrastructure for retirement protection; no medical and health insurance schemes in place to fund the aged care expenditures, leading to a reliance on taxation; and
6. Increasing pressure and burden on public funds in providing care for the elderly.

There are many indicators that successive Hong Kong governments' responses to aging of the population have been too late and too slow, and it remains to be seen if progress can now be made on the scale required. While acknowledging that community support services are the cornerstone of a successful policy for aging-in-place, the government stipulates that care for the elderly should remain the responsibility of the family. As a result, the development of community support services has lagged behind, and such services are a very small component in terms of the quantity of care services provided. Less than 1% of older persons were receiving in-home services in 1998 (Chi, Lam, & Chan, 1998).

There are severe shortages in community support services; for example, home help teams designed to serve 70 clients are on average serving 90 clients, an excess of close to 30%. Frail elderly may have to wait three months for urgently needed in-home services, and they may have no choice but to be admitted to an institution.

Although most elderly persons prefer to stay in their homes, almost 5% of those over 60 are living in some form of residential care providing various levels of care (Chi & Chow, 1997). More specifically, the proportion of the population aged 70 years and over in nursing homes is also 5%. These levels of use of residential care are comparable to western countries, and the high level of demand for residential care of different kinds is of considerable concern in Hong Kong's society, which upholds traditional Chinese values.

Both government and service providers are now expressing concerns about a number of common issues facing the future of long-term care:

1. Inadequate services to meet the demands, poor service matching, and no prioritization of service recipients.
2. Poor service coordination, which leads to service overlapping and fragmentation problems.
3. No standardized assessment/admission and referral/discharge criteria.
4. Poor service integration among health, nursing, and personal social services.
5. No quality control over services.
6. Limitations in funding sources.

TOWARDS A LONG-TERM CARE SYSTEM IN HONG KONG

Since 1997, the government has been calling for proposals to address the issues cited above. Several consultancy studies were commissioned to review the existing services, and most of the studies stipulated that there was an urgent need for developing an integrated service system. In 1998, a research team from the University of Hong Kong submitted a report to government that recommended the development of a new long-term care system (Chi, Lam, & Chan, 1998).

Since "long-term care" is not a familiar term in Hong Kong, the University consultancy first defined long-term care as: a continuum of health and social services delivered to clients with various levels of chronic health-related problems and/or disabilities on a long-term basis. It further recognized that elderly clients with long-term care needs will require care services from a continuum across different jurisdictions, agencies, and professional disciplines. Elderly clients eligible for long-term care were defined as having the following characteristics: frail with functional disabilities, incapable of self-care, medically stable, and in need of multiple services.

As a basis for developing Hong Kong's long-term care services into a *system* made up of a network of organizations that could provide a coordinated continuum of services to a defined population and that could be held clinically and fiscally responsible for the outcomes of the health status of the population served, the University consultancy identified the following core values:

- Care is provided in the most appropriate and efficient manner;
- Services are coordinated according to clients' and caregivers' needs;
- Choices of clients are respected;
- Care is provided using an evidence-based practice model; and
- Quality of life and care are maintained and/or enhanced.

The University consultancy team made a total of 18 recommendations. The nine recommendations that focused on building system infrastructure through integration, role differentiation, and improved quality of care, and the three on financing are noted in this article. The six recommendations on aspects of service delivery are taken up in the article, "Changing Needs and Changing Service Delivery for Long-Term Care in Hong Kong."

System Integration

A new Long-Term Care Office responsible for service coordination, service quality monitoring, and service funding was to be set up, preferably as a semi-government organization, functioning independently from the current government structure but reporting to government. The purpose of the Office was to coordinate, monitor quality, and fund long-term care services currently under government jurisdiction, but the Office would not offer direct services other than for reasons of efficiency and specialization of care required. Rather than a separate Office eventuating, however, the coordination, monitoring, and funding of long-term care have become focus areas within the Bureau of Health and Welfare, and outside specialists have been engaged to assist in setting out the agenda for long-term care planning.

Integration of all existing long-term-care-related services was recommended, to be achieved by realignment into four subsystems of acute and sub-acute geriatric services, residential care, community care, and home care. The new Long-Term Care Office was then to have varying levels of responsibility depending on the level of integration of services within each subsystem. It was to have full responsibility for services that were totally integrated in terms of eligibility criteria, service processes, administration, and funding; for services that were partially integrated, the Office was to be responsible for functions other than funding; and for minimally integrated services, it would be responsible only for eligibility criteria and service processes. As the new Office has not been established, progress towards integration has been slower than it might have been.

A shared governance structure was recommended, with a Long-Term Care Committee established at central level with membership made up of representatives from various stakeholders and client representatives. At the regional level, Long-Term Care Networks were to be established with regional representatives of various stakeholders, such as consumers, service partners, service contractors, and regional long-term care offices. Again, these committees have not emerged as separate entities but have been developed within existing administrative structures.

Role Differentiation

A general recommendation for clear role differentiation between service assessment and providers responsible for direct services was supported by two further recommendations: for the development of a *comprehensive assessment tool* to confirm eligibility for service, determine the appropriate level of care, and generate an appropriate care plan within available resources; and *specification of clear admission and discharge criteria, referral, and transfer arrangements*. There has been substantial progress with this set of recommendations: A standardized assessment is carried out by Long-Term Care Officers who have access to a regional Long-Term Care Consultant Team consisting of nursing, rehabilitation, and social work consultants. The standardized tool is the basis for client classification and funding.

A new mix of contractual relationships was to be developed to differentiate various types of service providers as partnerships or contractors with the Long-Term Care Office. Both forms of contract were to cover the overall responsibilities and accountabilities of both parties with respect to designated long-term care services, but providing for different funding arrangements. Even without the new Office, the government has achieved more variety in service agreements with service providers and in modes of funding.

Quality Measures

An inter-professional Practice Council was recommended to be established in each region to resolve disputes, consisting of representatives from health and social service professionals, and also having a role in promoting clinical practice standards. While this Council has not been implemented to date, the Social Welfare Department has established new inter-professional teams at the regional level to carry out the standardized assessments.

A quality management program was recommended at the onset of the new system. It was to specify clear indicators for long-term care outcomes, including health status, clients'/caregivers' experiences, process efficiency, innovation/learning, and cost, and to have a comprehensive management strategy, including monitoring, quality improvement, and quality planning. This program was also expected to add confidence to all stakeholders including clients, the general public, and service providers. The quality management program was not to be an add-on responsibility, but rather the responsibility of each employee and agency in the system. Although a comprehensive quality management program has not been implemented, progress is evident, most notably in the requirements for service providers participating in the Enhanced Home Care Program to provide information on quality indicators and outcome measures, for both clinical and management areas.

Financing

Expansion of the private care market was recommended to address the needs of long-term care clients who could afford to purchase services. Historically, all long-term care services have been funded by government and delivered through the non-governmental agencies, and many private nursing homes are funded indirectly since their residents are public assistance recipients. There are very few private agencies providing community-based or in-home services such as homemaking, personal care, and nursing services in Hong Kong. The private market homemaking services are more flexible than the subvented services and do not have waiting lists; they are less rigid in terms of using part-time workers, and less constrained by geographic boundaries. While these services charge a reasonable rate and are able to compete with subvented services, they cannot compete with the imported labor employed as live-in maids. Although opportunities have been opened for more private provision of long-term care services, the scale of the market for fully self-financed services appears small and is having some difficulty surviving.

User fees were recommended as a further stimulus to the private market and as a stimulus to competition with the subvented sector. At present, there is a division between subsidized services in the subvented sector, with very low fees regardless of income, and private services, which are full-cost recovery (with the exception of the "bought beds" scheme). Adoption of means testing could divert some clients from subvented services to the private market, but the government has not gone so far as offering to subsidize the private sector to cater to low-income clients.

Finally, it was recommended that the government should begin to explore the introduction of a long-term care insurance scheme in Hong Kong by making reference to other developed countries. There would be many implementation considerations if this recommendation were adopted, particularly whether public health insurance, if introduced in Hong Kong, would also cover long-term care, or whether private health insurance should be encouraged to launch long-term care products in the market. The present priority is with the implementation of a provident fund scheme for retirement savings, and any action on health or long-term care insurance will have to wait until the outcomes of this initiative are seen.

The Agenda in Action

The recommendations made by the University consultancy set out an agenda for the government, and its preparedness to take a leadership role and to make the commitment to long-term care is evident in the action taken to date. The University consultancy also recognized that since most of the service providers in Hong Kong were not familiar with the concepts or practice of an integrated long-term care system, changes would need to be introduced gradually and implemented steadily, with improved communication between service providers and funding organizations, and more educational opportunities.

In the short term, attention has focused on establishing the infrastructure necessary to improve the elderly services in Hong Kong, to increase efficiency, and to encourage integration and collaboration among the professionals. The medium term should see the cumulative effects of these policy and planning measures interact with progress in service delivery. Securing funding sources and implementing effective quality control measures remain to be addressed in the longer term.

REFERENCES

Census and Statistics Department (1998). *The Report on Elderly Population*. Hong Kong: Hong Kong Government Printing Office.
Chi, I., & Chow, N. S. W. (1997). Housing and Family Care of the Elderly People in Hong Kong. *Aging International, Winter/Spring:* 65-77.

Chi, I., & Chui, E. (1999). Ageing in Hong Kong. *Australasian Journal on Ageing*, *18*(2): 66-71.

Chi, I., Lam, Z., & Chan, P. (1998). *Consultancy Report on Community Support Services for the Elderly People in Hong Kong.* Hong Kong: The University of Hong Kong.

Chi, I., & Lee, J. J. (1991). Health Education for the Elderly in Hong Kong. *Educational Gerontology*, *17*(5): 507-516.

Chiu, H., Lam, L., Chi, I., & Pang, A. (1998). An Epidemiological Study of Dementia in the Elderly in Hong Kong. *Neurology*, *50*:1002-1009.

Harvard Report (1999). *Improving Hong Kong's Health Care System: Why and for Whom?* Hong Kong: Government Printing Office.

Hong Kong Government (1997). *Policy Address by the Chief Executive.* Hong Kong: Government Printing Office.

Hong Kong Government (1999). *Policy Address by the Chief Executive.* Hong Kong: Government Printing Office.

Social Welfare Department (1997). *Annual Report.* Hong Kong: Government Printing Office.

Social Welfare Department (1999). *Five-Year Plan.* Hong Kong: Government Printing Office.

Social Welfare Department (2000). *Annual Report.* Hong Kong: Government Printing Office.

Yip, P., Chi, I., & Yu, K. K. (1998). An Epidemiological Profile of Elderly Suicide in Hong Kong. *International Journal of Geriatric Psychiatry*, *13*: 631-637.

Changing Needs
and Changing Service Delivery
for Long-Term Care in Hong Kong

Edward M. F. Leung, FRCP

President, Hong Kong Association of Gerontology
Consultant Geriatrician, United Christian Hospital, Hong Kong

SUMMARY. Both the need for and delivery of long-term care in Hong Kong are shaped by the interaction of the traditional and modern. Rapid social change is affecting traditional family structures and roles in care of the elderly, resulting in increased demand for formal care, which to date has been provided mainly by way of residential care. This growth of

Dr. Edward M. F. Leung, FHKAM (Medicine), FRCP (Edinburgh, London, Glasgow), is President, Hong Kong Association of Gerontology and Chief of Service, Department of Medicine and Geriatrics, United Christian Hospital, Hong Kong. He was graduated from the Faculty of Medicine, University of Hong Kong in 1979 and has been working in the field of Geriatric Medicine since 1980. He received his MRCP (UK) in 1985, FRCP (Edinburgh) in 1994, FRCP (London) and FRCP (Glasgow) in 2000, and is also a Fellow of the Hong Kong Academy of Medicine and the Hong Kong College of Physicians. His major research interests are epidemiology in old age, health promotion, osteoporosis, fall, stroke, incontinence, long-term care, and public policy in old age. Dr. Leung has published widely in local and international journals and has been a contributor to a number of books on health and aging. He has been an invited keynote speaker at symposia in Korea, Japan, Singapore, Australia, China, and Taiwan.

Dr. Leung can be contacted at the Department of Medicine and Geriatrics, United Christian Hospital, 130 Hip Wo St., Kwan Tong, Kowloon, Hong Kong (E-mail: emfleung@ha.org.hk).

[Haworth co-indexing entry note]: "Changing Needs and Changing Service Delivery for Long-Term Care in Hong Kong ." Leung, Edward M. F. Co-published simultaneously in *Journal of Aging & Social Policy* (The Haworth Press, Inc.) Vol. 13, No. 2/3, 2001, pp. 155-168; and: *Long-Term Care in the 21st Century: Perspectives from Around the Asia-Pacific Rim* (ed: Iris Chi, Kalyani K. Mehta, and Anna L. Howe) The Haworth Press, Inc., 2001, pp. 155-168. Single or multiple copies of this article are available for a fee from The Haworth Document Delivery Service [1-800-HAWORTH, 9:00 a.m. - 5:00 p.m. (EST). E-mail address: getinfo@haworthpressinc.com].

155

demand will escalate with rapid population aging in coming decades. In response to this burgeoning demand, current planning is seeking to re-shape the established service system and tackle problems in service delivery in ways that will address the bias towards residential care and improve quality of care. *[Article copies available for a fee from The Haworth Document Delivery Service: 1-800-HAWORTH. E-mail address: <getinfo@haworthpressinc.com> Website: <http://www.HaworthPress.com> © 2001 by The Haworth Press, Inc. All rights reserved.]*

KEYWORDS. Chronic illness, family roles, Hong Kong, quality, residential care

THE NEED FOR CARE

Two main factors shape the need for long-term care in Hong Kong, and both will bring changes in need in the next decade. First, rapid aging of the population is bringing an increase in the number of older persons who may suffer from ill health and disabilities, resulting in the need for care and support by others. Second, and more particular to Hong Kong, is the effect of rapid change in family structures and support. In the past, when the traditional extended family was in place, care of the older relatives was in the hands of their younger family members, especially the women. With increasing standards of living, and increasing costs, it is the norm for family size to be reduced and for women to participate in the paid labor force. The capacity of the family to look after older parents is thus reduced.

The need for long-term care in Hong Kong can be examined from three dimensions: defining the population at risk, developing a profile of people in need of long-term care, and the system of service delivery. To prepare for the challenge of population aging in Hong Kong, the need for long-term care in the population must be assessed, and the problems of delivery of long-term care services must be identified. To tackle these problems, strategic directions for future development need to be developed. Accordingly, this paper examines the need for long-term care, problems of delivery, and future directions of long-term care in Hong Kong.

Defining Population Need

The term "long-term care" has been defined by Kane as "Care delivered to individuals who are dependent on others for assistance with the basic task necessary for physical, mental, and social functioning over sustained period of time" (Kane & Kane, 1989). Following this definition, the size of the long-term care problem in Hong Kong can be examined in terms of the potential number of people who may be in need of long-term care on the basis of potential support and health status.

Indicators of Support. Traditionally, informal care shouldered the major part of long-term care as elderly people with mild disabilities could usually be cared for by family members at home. However, many of those who are living alone or living with their spouses only are potentially in need of long-term care when their health condition deteriorates and disability sets in. Results of the 1991 Census set out in Table 1 show that 11% of elderly people in Hong Kong were living alone, and 12% were living with their spouse only; another 8% were living with unrelated persons. It is estimated that 31% of elderly people in Hong Kong are at risk of having insufficient support once their health conditions deteriorate.

Marital status of the elderly population is also important in predicting the strength of support likely to be available to them. As seen in Table 2, the 1991 Census showed that 5% of the elderly population were never married, and 65% were still married. Another 29% were widowed, with widowhood being almost four times more common among women than men, and a small minority were divorced or separated. The large group of elderly widows stands out as the group with potentially limited family support, and the need for long-term care poses a serious problem for this group.

Health Status. Apart from the extent and strength of the caring network of the family, health status and prevalence of disabling diseases in the elderly population are important predictors of the need for long-term care in Hong Kong. A number of studies have provided evidence that the prevalence of chronic illnesses amongst elderly people in Hong Kong is high (Chi & Lee, 1989; Leung & Lo, 1997). For example, a recent community health survey has shown that chronic degenerative diseases, like diabetes, hypertension, and stroke, were more common among elderly people compared with the younger adult population (Leung & Lau, 1999). Figures in Table 3 show that the rates of these conditions among the 65 and over age group were more than double the rates for the 40-64 age group. Rates of chronic illness were also higher for women than men in both the middle age and older age groups.

Another study among 1,480 elderly people living in the community found that chronic illnesses were common, increasing with age, and more so among women. Almost one in three had a diagnosis of either rheumatism or hypertension, and almost one in five had sustained a fracture. A wide range of other chronic and disabling complaints were diagnosed for at least 5% of the population, including peptic ulcer (13.5%), diabetes mellitus (10.7%), chronic bronchitis (8.2%), coronary heart disease (6.8%), hyperthyroidism (6.1%), and

TABLE 1. Living Arrangements of Elderly Population, by Age, Hong Kong Census, 1991

Living Arrangements	Age Group				Total	
	60-64	65-74	75-84	85 and over	Number	%
Alone	17,536	33,345	19,098	3,184	73,163	10.9
Spouse only	26,339	41,262	13,245	1,077	81,923	12.2
Children only	22,136	30,103	8,983	1,571	62,821	9.3
Spouse & Children	86,990	71,836	11,621	527	170,974	25.4
Other Persons	11,864	21,639	14,662	4,038	52,203	7.8
Spouse & Others	5,724	9,302	3,340	347	18,713	2.8
Children & Other	20,788	52,618	34,044	9,502	116,952	17.4
Spouse & Children & Other Persons	37,098	45,363	12,782	1,204	96,447	14.3
Total	228,475	305,496	117,775	21,450	673,196	100

Source: Hong Kong Government (1994).

TABLE 2. Marital Status of Population Aged 60 and Over by Sex, Hong Kong Census, 1991

Marital Status	Male		Female		Total	
	No.	%	No.	%	No.	%
Never Married	16,665	5.0	17,021	4.4	33,686	4.7
Married	271,308	81.7	191,806	49.9	463,114	64.6
Widowed	39,382	11.9	170,243	44.2	209,625	29.2
Divorced/Separated	47,861	1.4	5,690	1.5	10,476	1.5
Total	332,141	100.0	384,760	100.0	716,901	100.0

Source: Hong Kong Government (1994).

stroke (3.8%). In the same study, 12% of the elderly were found to have three or more impairments in activities of daily living, indicating their need for personal assistance at home.

In addition to physical conditions and functional disabilities, cognitive impairment, especially dementia, is an important predictor of need for long-term care. According to a 1993 study by Liu, 11% of elderly people over the age of 65 have an impairment of cognitive function as measured by the Mini-Mental

State Examination. As seen in Table 4, the prevalence of cognitive impairment increased rapidly after the age of 80, reaching 26% of those aged above 80. These findings show levels of cognitive impairment comparable to most other studies in developed countries (Liu, 1993).

EXPRESSED DEMAND FOR LONG-TERM CARE

Conventionally, the provision of formal long-term care services in Hong Kong has mainly been provided through residential services, which are of

TABLE 3. Chronic Diseases by Age and Sex, 1996

% reporting by diagnosis	Age							
	<18		18-39		40-64		65 and over	
	Male	Female	Male	Female	Male	Female	Male	Female
Back Pain	0.4	0	0.4	1.4	9.5	13.0	24.9	34.5
Hypertension	0	0	0.4	0.6	7.2	12.4	17.8	26.9
Rheumatism	0.2	0.2	1.3	2.2	6.9	7.8	7.5	14.1
Diabetes	0	0	0	0.2	2.2	4.9	6.1	12.0
Chronic Bronchitis	0.4	0.2	0.2	0.7	0.3	1.8	3.8	2.4
Heart Disease	0	0	0.1	0.1	0.8	1.8	3.8	5.6
Stroke	0	0	0	0	0.3	0	3.8	1.6

Source: Leung & Lau (1999).

TABLE 4. Status of Cognitive Function of Persons Over Age 65

Gender	% of sample (n = 2203)	% with MMSE	
		< = 20	20+
Male	45.6	6.5	93.5
Female	54.4	15.1	84.9
	100.0	11.2	88.8
Age			
65-69	41.2	5.7	94.3
70-74	29.4	11.1	88.9
75-79	18.4	14.7	85.3
80+	11.0	26.0	74.0

Source: Liu et al. (1993).

three types: care and attention homes in the not-for-profit sector, infirmaries in public hospitals, and care homes in the private sector. The levels of care provided in these homes range from basic support to full nursing care.

Current Levels of Use

The number of people currently residing in these homes and the growth of such homes in recent years provide indicators of the demand for residential care. Apart from government supported care and attention homes and infirmaries, people in need of long-term care can also obtain services from private residential homes that provide services for elderly people with varying care needs. The number of people residing in private homes serves as a good indicator of the demand for long-term care. In 1998 there were 22,000 private residential home beds, and the number has been increasing in the past few years. Adding all residential places together, more than 32,000 elderly people were in residential care institutions in Hong Kong in 1997 (Table 5), accounting for 5% of the total population aged 65 and over. About one third of all residential care places were in institutions providing a nursing home level of care, including infirmaries, subvented nursing homes, places in care and attention homes in the subvented sector that received a nursing home supplement, and dementia care units.

The profile of residents in nursing homes shows a highly dependent population. Two separate surveys of private nursing homes (Leung, J. Y. Y. et al., 2000; Sim & Leung, E. M. F., 2000) found that the average age of residents was 80 years, and that 70% were female. Indicators of dependency reported in both studies showed that approximately 30% were chair- or bed bound, 40% had urinary or bowel incontinence, and between 20% and 30% were taking more than five medications. Both studies also raised concerns about frequent admissions of private nursing home patients to acute hospitals and the lack of an effective presence of geriatric medical services in these nursing homes.

Waiting Lists

A further indication of expressed demand for long-term care services can be gained from the number of people applying for institutional care each year, which appear on the government-maintained waiting list. The number of elderly people on the waiting lists for care and attention homes increased from 11,228 in 1994 to 19,278 in 1998, an increase of 72%, and for infirmaries from 5,964 in 1994 to 7,171 in 1998, an increase of 20%. As of 1998, some 26,000 older people had expressed a demand for residential care.

TABLE 5. Growth of Long-Term Care Facilities in Hong Kong, 1993-1997

Year	Subvented Sector Care & Attention Homes	Public Sector Infirmary Beds	Private Sector Care Homes
1993	3,789	1,128	14,787
1994	5,539	1,203	17,269
1995	6,745	1,472	20,698
1996	8,169	1,772	22,978
1997	8,829	1,915	22,800
Increase 1993-97	133%	70%	54%

Source: Leung (2000).

These figures indicate that the growth of demand is well ahead of the growth of the aged population, but some of the demand comes from individuals in private homes seeking alternative places in subsidized care and attention homes in the subvented sector. No figures on waiting lists are available for private homes, but the increase in provision noted above indicates similar growth of demand, and a study by Ngan et al. (1996) demonstrated that a significant number of people on the waiting list for places in public facilities had already obtained services from private residential homes.

Profile of Elderly People in Need of Long-Term Care

Since the government established the waiting list for residential services for elderly people in Hong Kong in the early 1990s, studies of the profile of elderly people on these lists have provided further information on the potential demand of long-term care in the future. The study by Ngan et al. (1996) demonstrated that those elderly people in need of long-term residential care have higher prevalence of chronic and disabling diseases in comparison to the general population. Results reported in Table 6 show that higher percentages of those on the infirmary waiting lists had dementia or suffered a stroke, with stroke being a major factor precipitating need for long-term care.

PROVISION OF LONG-TERM CARE

While the provision of long-term care in Hong Kong can be divided into institutional and community care, the resources put in place in the past have been geared mainly towards residential care. The components of institutional long-

TABLE 6. Prevalence of Chronic Illnesses in Elderly on Waiting Lists for Residential Care

Diagnosis	% reporting diagnosis on waiting list for	
	Infirmary	Care & Attention Home
Stroke	43.1	21.5
Dementia	24.8	4.3
Hypertension	22.5	28.4
Diabetes	15.0	20.1
Other Fractures	6.8	7.0
Fracture Femur	7.5	5.2
Parkinsonism	7.5	2.6

Source: Ngan, Leung et al. (1996)

term care in Hong Kong include aged care homes, care and attention homes, and nursing homes.

Due to their historical pattern of development, the subvented homes are classified into different types on the basis of the level of frailty of residents and care provided, and residents may have to move if their level of care changes. Aged care homes provide communal living accommodation for those elderly persons who, though capable of self-care, are psychologically in need of support and supervision in their daily lives. Services include meals and laundry, very limited personal care, and social activities. Care and attention homes provide accommodation with general personal care and limited nursing care for elderly people who suffer from poor health or physical/mental disabilities. The higher cost of the care and attention homes comes from the higher level of services, which include regular medical, nursing, and rehabilitative services, social support, and personal care. The nursing homes in the subvented sector provide an even higher level of skilled nursing care.

Private homes cover all levels of care and have adopted a continuum of care model, admitting residents at varying levels of frailty. Payment for "bought places" in private homes varies according to the level of care provided. Private homes that rely on income from residents' fees are polarized between those providing very basic support to residents receiving CSSA and those providing high levels and standards of care to the small number of elderly people who can afford considerably higher fees.

Fewer resources are allocated to community support for elderly people in need of long-term care than are allocated to institutional care. As a result, community care for frail elderly people is relatively underdeveloped. In the past few years, the Hong Kong government has become aware of the importance of community support for the frail elderly, and a number of community-based programs have been developed. Such programs include: community geriatric assessment teams, community nursing services, home help, meals delivery, day care, respite, and caregiver support. Furthermore, since 1999, the Hong Kong SAR government has developed a number of new initiatives to improve the quality of long-term care for elderly people in community and residential homes. Specifically, the initiatives have directed attention to quality of care in the provision of dementia care, better assessment, and developing the continuum of care in residential homes.

The development of elderly services in Hong Kong has been based mainly on services in the United Kingdom. The spectrum of long-term care services is distributed across a wide range of different providers, including government departments and non-government organizations. The governmental agencies involved in long-term care include the Hong Kong Hospital Authority and Social Welfare Department; non-governmental organizations include volunteers, neighborhood support groups, and family caregivers.

PROBLEMS IN PROVIDING LONG-TERM CARE

Problems affecting the provision of long-term care for elderly people in Hong Kong include high, unmet demand, changes in family structure and expectations of the role of the government in support of elderly people, and problems in the service delivery structure.

High, Unmet Demand

The high demand for long-term care institutions in Hong Kong has already been discussed. There has been a significant increase in the number of people aged 75 years and older on the wait list for community-based care. This high, unmet demand has resulted in the proliferation of private care homes that are largely unregulated. In many cases, poor standards in such homes contribute to the deteriorating health status of elderly people admitted to them.

Weakening of Family Care

There is an increasing trend for elderly people in Hong Kong to live alone or with their spouses only. The traditional three-generation household and extended family structure has become a rarity in Hong Kong. With the high cost of living rising, women are increasingly required to work to support family expenses. This trend contributes to the weakening of support for frail elderly people, even in a traditional family where grandparents are living with their children's family but are exposed to the risk of failing care and support due to their family members' need to work out of the home.

The change of political status of Hong Kong in 1997 was preceded by a wave of out-migration of younger people during the 1980s and 1990s, resulting in further disruption of family structures and caring networks. In some cases, elderly parents have been left alone in Hong Kong and therefore applied for residential homes. The burden of care has been left to the adult children remaining in Hong Kong.

With westernized education and urban living styles, the community expectation on the role of family and government has undergone tremendous changes. Family members increasingly turn to government support when their parents become frail and in need of care. This has contributed to the rapidly increasing demand for care homes in Hong Kong.

Problems in the Delivery System

Long-term care institutions have relied heavily on funding from government, and there are no alternative funding mechanisms apart from out-of-pocket expenditures. The concept of medical insurance is underdeveloped in Hong Kong, and long-term care insurance is essentially non-existent. The limited sources of funding have severely affected the market's ability to respond to the high need for long-term care. Frail elderly people requiring care are mostly accommodated in institutions, and the high degree of institutionalization is a direct consequence of an underdeveloped community support system. One indicator of this imbalance is the minimal utilization of respite care in Hong Kong.

Hong Kong has been mainly concerned with meeting more long-standing problems than with providing post-acute care as occurs in the United States. In Hong Kong, after an elderly person experiences a catastrophic acute event such as a major stroke, the family must provide care until a proper placement is available.

A final problem in the delivery of long-term care is that the various types of institutional and community services are divided between multiple providers in medical and welfare settings, and cooperation between them has long been problematic. Furthermore, quality of service varies among providers.

ISSUES FOR THE FUTURE

Meeting the Need for Long-Term Care

To meet the rising need of long-term care in Hong Kong, measures must first be implemented to help the most needy. With implementation of needs assessment and frequent monitoring of population trends, prediction of future care needs will be improved. To this end, there is the need to define the population at risk. A needs-related planning mechanism, based on systematic collection of epidemiological trends and feedback from assessment of the elderly population, would enable better planning for the provision of long-term care.

Modes of Delivery

A number of the problems in service delivery are structural. The spread of providers across the welfare and hospital sectors has created misunderstanding and fragmentation of services. In addition, funding for long-term care has mainly been provided to operators, not elderly people. This has resulted in residential homes' preferring to admit the less disabled and those requiring less intensive care. To improve the delivery of long-term care, a needs-related funding system, possibly of a voucher type, would encourage operators to look after elderly people with all kinds of needs.

The entry point to obtaining long-term care in Hong Kong can be confusing: elderly people and their caregivers often need to go to several agencies to obtain various services such as day care, home help, and day hospitals. The creation of a single point of entry to the service system would enhance the accessibility, and steps to this end are in progress. In September 2000, the Social Welfare Department established a Standard Care Need Assessment Mechanism Office to provide a central point for the standard assessment of elderly people in need of long-term care services, including residential services and community-based services. Such standardized assessment can help to redress the practice of referring long-term care recipients to services at various agencies (Hong Kong Government, 2000).

The current funding to residential homes according to number of beds gives no recognition to the level of dependency and frailty of residents. An effective classification system for long-term care recipients would help to delineate the needs of recipients in various long-term care settings. Resident classification instruments that have been well developed in other countries such as Australia and the United States can provide a guide for development in Hong Kong.

The bias towards residential care and the underdevelopment of community support and rehabilitation services must be addressed to improve the provision of long-term care to elderly people, and more comprehensive and accessible community care options should be made available. Attention should also be given to caregiver support and the role of women in caring for their family members, with community services geared towards relieving caregiver burden.

Advocacy for Recipients of Long-Term Care

Elderly people in need of long-term care are often unable to defend their own rights. An ombudsman could play an important role in protecting the well-being of older people receiving long-term care services. At this time, there are no Ombudsman Services in Hong Kong.

DIRECTIONS FOR THE FUTURE

Facing a rapid increase in the old-old population, strengthening community care has been identified as the main direction for the future of service delivery in Hong Kong. The attention to community care reflects not only concerns about the growth of residential care, but a more fundamental recognition of changes in family structures that generate a need for extended support to enhance the capacity of families to care for frail elderly family members. In future, the balance between informal care and formal services will see more formal community services supporting informal care by the family.

The framework through which formal community services development is occurring has been shaped by the University of Hong Kong consultancy, which reported to the government in 1998 (Chi, Lam, & Chan, 1998). As well as making recommendations on policy and planning, as discussed in "Long-Term Care Policy for Elders in Hong Kong," six recommendations addressed critical aspects of community care.

Comprehensive Care Planning

Care planning for individual clients was recommended as an essential link between assessment and coordination of service delivery. A care-management approach was recommended to implement services in accord with the levels recommended on assessment by the Long-Term Care Consultation Teams. Involvement of family caregivers in care planning was also recognized.

Components of Long-Term Care

To protect the well-being of frail elderly people, a full range of long-term care services should include the mix of institutional and community-based facilities and programs. The consultancy identified three areas as priorities to extend the range of community services in Hong Kong. First, an enhanced community-living program was recommended, providing integrated social and rehabilitative day activities to reduce isolation and to support long-term care clients who require ongoing home support. Second, a number of measures were proposed to increase the efficiency of delivered meals services, to foster innovations such as group dining integrated with social and recreational activities, and to improve nutritional standards. Third, attention was called to the need to ensure that the nursing component of home care was adequate to address the increasing complexity of long-term care clients' needs.

Workforce Development and Training

An essential requirement for the provision of long-term care services is that the workers involved have the necessary knowledge and skills. While well-trained health care professionals with specialist skills in aged care are established in Hong Kong, including geriatricians, nurses, social workers, and rehabilitation professionals, the major part of care and assistance in the community is provided by unskilled or semi-skilled workers. To complement the recommendation for increased use of trained nursing staff in community care, a recommendation was made for the provision of additional training to enhance the skills of home care and home help staff.

The second recommendation in the area of workforce development was for the increased use of volunteer services in tasks associated with day programs, such as escorting and meal delivery. The need for volunteer training and coordination by professionals and volunteer organizations was recognized. The provision of training to family caregivers is also important in reducing their stress and burden in day-to-day care of elderly parents.

Commitment to the Enhanced Home Care Program

Perhaps the most concrete evidence of commitment to expanding community care and strengthening its part in service delivery is the establishment of the Enhanced Home Care Program. The allocation of $HK68m for this program in 2001-02 has met a very ready response with over 60 non-government providers submitting applications to participate. Since April 2001, this program has supported one program per district to deliver in-home health and social care to frail elders who have been assessed and who are either waiting for residential care or are eligible for residential care but prefer to remain at home.

As well as having an immediate effect in the short term, the Enhanced Home Care Program provides a firm foundation on which integrated community care can be built in the future. As well as initiating standardized assessment and improved care planning and management, the Enhanced Home Care Program will extend the range of services provided. A stronger community care system will in turn strengthen and be strengthened by opportunities for workforce development. Along with other policy measures addressing contractual and funding relationships between providers and government, the stage is set for the quality community care to be realized in the delivery of long-term care in Hong Kong in the first decade of the 21st century.

REFERENCES

Chi, I., Lam, Z. & Chan, P. (1998). *Consultancy Report on Community Support Services for the Elderly People in Hong Kong.* Hong Kong: The University of Hong Kong.

Chi, I., & Lee, J. J. (1989). *A Health Survey of the Elderly in Hong Kong.* Department of Social Work and Social Administration, University of Hong Kong.

Chi, I., & Chow, N. (1997). Housing and family care for the elderly in Hong Kong. *Ageing International,* Winter/Spring: 65-77.

Hong Kong Government (2000). Policy Address, Hong Kong: Government Printer.

Kane, R. L., & Kane, R. A. (1989). Transitions in long-term care, in Ory, M. G. & Bond, K. (Eds.). *Ageing and Health Care: Social Science and Policy Perspectives.* London: Routledge.

Leung, E. M. F., & Lo, M. B. N. (1997). Social and health status of elderly people in Hong Kong, in Lam, S. K. (Ed.). *The Health of the Elderly in Hong Kong.* Hong Kong: Hong Kong University Press.

Leung, E. M. F., & Lau, J. T. F. (1999). *Report on Survey of Health Care Needs in Kwun Tong.* Hong Kong: United Christian Hospital.

Leung, E. M. F. (2000). Long term care issues in the Asia-Pacific region, in Phillips (Ed.). *Ageing in the Asia Pacific Region.* London: Routledge.

Leung, J. Y. Y., Yu, T. K. K., Cheung, Y. L., Ma., L. C., Cheung, S. P., & Wong, C. P. (2000). Private nursing home residents in Hong Kong–How frail are they and their need for hospital services. *Journal of the Hong Kong Geriatric Society, 10*(2): 65-69.

Liu, W. T., Lee, R. P. L., Yu, E. S. H., Lee, J. J., & Sun, S. G. (1993). *Health Status, Cognitive Functioning and Dementia among Elderly Community Population in Hong Kong.* Hong Kong: Hong Kong Baptist College

Ngan, R. M. H., Leung, E. M. F., Kwan, A. Y. H., Yeung, D. W. T., & Chong, A. M. L. (1996). *A Study of Long-Term Care Needs, Pattern and Impact of the Elderly in Hong Kong.* Hong Kong: City University of Hong Kong.

Sim, T. C., & Leung, E. M. F. (2000). Geriatric care for residents of private nursing homes. *Journal of the Hong Kong Geriatrics Society, 10*(2): 84-89.

The Savings Approach to Financing Long-Term Care in Singapore

Phua Kai Hong, PhD

National University of Singapore

SUMMARY. Singapore is grappling with provision of services for the current generation of older people at the same time as building the foundation for the coming generations of elderly. In this article, I analyze four sets of factors that are shaping long-term care policy and financing in ways that are almost unique to Singapore. First, current developments can only be understood in the context of the Central Provident Fund (CPF) that was established by the Government of Singapore in the 1950s to ensure that the working population saved for retirement; the Medisave and related schemes for financing health care were subsequently developed alongside the CPF. Most recently, the existing funding arrangements have been extended to some long-term care services, and options

Dr. Phua Kai Hong is Associate Professor of Health Policy and Management, and Director of Health Services Research at the Department of Community, Occupational, and Family Medicine, National University of Singapore. Dr. Hong has been appointed to many national advisory committees, including the Government Parliamentary Committee Resource Panel on Health (1988-1996), the National Advisory Council on the Family and Aged (1989-1994), and the Review Committee on National Health Policies (1991-1992). He is presently appointed as Resource Person to the Workgroup on Health Care and Chairman of the Sub-Workgroup on Resource Funding, in the Inter-Ministerial Committee on the Ageing Population.

Dr. Hong can be contacted at the Dept. of Community, Occupational, and Family Medicine, MD 3, National University of Singapore, 10 Kent Ridge Crescent, Singapore 119260 (E-mail: cofpkh@nus.edu.sg).

[Haworth co-indexing entry note]: "The Savings Approach to Financing Long-Term Care in Singapore." Hong, Phua Kai. Co-published simultaneously in *Journal of Aging & Social Policy* (The Haworth Press, Inc.) Vol. 13, No. 2/3, 2001, pp. 169-183; and: *Long-Term Care in the 21st Century: Perspectives from Around the Asia-Pacific Rim* (ed: Iris Chi, Kalyani K. Mehta, and Anna L. Howe) The Haworth Press, Inc., 2001, pp. 169-183. Single or multiple copies of this article are available for a fee from The Haworth Document Delivery Service [1-800-HAWORTH, 9:00 a.m. - 5:00 p.m. (EST). E-mail address: getinfo@haworthpressinc.com].

for further extensions are under consideration. Second, the government's philosophy of maintaining the primacy of family support for the elderly has been expressed through a number of initiatives that provide financial and other incentives to families, combined with an emphasis on community care. The third factor is the relationship between government and the voluntary welfare organizations that are the major providers of institutional and community services. Finally, a series of government-sponsored reviews and advisory councils have provided for widespread consultation on policy options. These developments are directed to achieving a multi-pillar approach in which intergenerational transfers through taxation will be limited, and the role of individual savings and insurance will be increased. *[Article copies available for a fee from The Haworth Document Delivery Service: 1-800-HAWORTH. E-mail address: <getinfo@haworthpressinc.com> Website: <http://www.HaworthPress.com> © 2001 by The Haworth Press, Inc. All rights reserved.]*

KEYWORDS. Central Provident Fund, family, financing, voluntary organizations, savings, Singapore

THE POLICY CONTEXT

Financing care for the aging population has surfaced as a critical issue in many Asian countries that are undergoing rapid demographic and epidemiological transitions. In Singapore, the rapid aging of the population is expected to intensify the demand for and expenditure on health care and long-term care, making it necessary to plan for appropriate and cost-effective services so that the organization and financing of long-term care can be integrated with arrangements for income support and health care to guard against the pressures of increasing costs. This paper presents an account of the integrated approach that is being taken to directing Singapore's policies towards achieving this objective.

The core measure for addressing aging in Singapore is the Central Provident Fund (CPF), which was set up in the 1950s as a universal, compulsory saving scheme to provide income support for the working population when they retired. The early development and operation of the CPF have been reported in detail by Sherraden (1970). Subsequent provisions for health care have been integrated with the CPF, and together these measures set the context in which arrangements for long-term care are now being developed. A Public Assistance scheme is administered by the Ministry of Community Development to provide a minimum income for the destitute, frail, and disabled elderly who have no income from their CPF accounts and no family support. While the issues of population aging faced by Singapore have much in common with other rapidly aging countries of the region, the initial solutions devised by way of the CPF and further elaborations building on that foundation have set in train a system that is in many ways unique to Singapore.

It is now almost 20 years since the Singapore government began to recognize the impact an aging population would have on society. In line with its philosophy of long-term planning and with some considerable foresight, the government set up an Inter-Ministerial Population Committee (IMC) in 1984. This was to be the first of a series of inter-ministerial committees that have examined issues of aging over the ensuing years. It should be noted that as retirement age in Singapore is 55 years, "the elderly," as used in this paper, refers to the population aged 55 and over; specific ages are identified in instances where reference is made to other age groups.

In 1988, the National Advisory Council on the Aged was formed to undertake a comprehensive review of the status of aging in Singapore. One of its key recommendations was that a National Council on Ageing should be set up with the character and authority of a statutory board to plan effectively and coordinate policies and programs for older persons. Proposals relating to retirement included raising the retirement age from 55 to 60 because continued employment would provide a sense of worth, dignity, and financial independence to older persons; and adjusting the seniority-based wage system to remove disincentives to employ more older people. Two proposals that recognized the value of old people in the community were made, one to expand and strengthen public education programs about older persons and aging so that positive attitudes towards older persons could be inculcated, and another to increase the dependency tax rebate for families who look after older persons. Proposals designed to contribute to service development were: to make land available for voluntary organizations to set up homes for older persons and to lengthen the terms of leases for these homes, to address the scarcity and high cost of land in Singapore, and to study the feasibility of providing health and medical services for the frail older persons living in their own homes.

A number of these initiatives have been acted on to support family care for the elderly and so give expression to the government's philosophy of maintaining family support. Measures taken include provision of financial incentives linked to CPF contributions and preferential treatment in allocation of housing and housing loans, closely integrated with the wider housing and income security policies that are particular to Singapore. These measures are reported to have increased the proportion of elderly living with family from 81% to 86% in 1995 (Lee, 1999). This 5% shift is more impressive when seen as a relative decline among the 19% of the elderly who were not previously living with their children because it indicates a change in living arrangements for one in four of this group. Allowing for the proportion of the elderly who have no children, family living arrangements are evidently being sustained.

To meet further challenges, the 1990s saw the development and implementation of three milestone policies. A significant piece of legislation, the Maintenance of Parents Act, was introduced in 1994 after extensive deliberation by various community groups and a Parliamentary Select Committee. The policy aims to prevent the neglect of elderly parents and to provide action when problems arise; public endorsement for this policy that imposes a legal obligation on children to maintain their parents is again quite particular to Singapore. In 1996, amendments to the Women's Charter provided channels for elderly parents to exercise legal action if they were victims of physical, mental, or psychological abuse. An enlightened policy covering medical care of the terminally ill was also put in place in 1996. Under the Advanced Medical Directive Act, persons who have been medically certified to be brain dead can now be relieved of medical life support. This policy is seen as reducing unnecessary suffering for both the terminally ill older persons and their families, but the present take-up rate is rather low, and it is not expected to play a significant role in the immediate future.

Beyond these specific initiatives, a national policy on aging in Singapore has taken shape after a number of policy reviews. Two characteristics in the policy formulation process have been noted. First, the various Committees have the benefit of representation from various sectors and so receive diverse input from government ministries and agencies, from providers, professional and community organizations, leading to decisions that are likely to be implemented. Historically, cross-sector representation has worked well in the local context, and it is a standard feature in Singapore's government problem-solving approach. Second, the Committees were given wide publicity, and public awareness of the issues of aging was heightened, especially when controversial recommendations were proposed. The enhanced discussion of policy changes by the public has seen an increasing emphasis on social care of older persons.

The most recent IMC on the Ageing Population, formed in 1998, has revisited many of the recommendations of earlier Committees on aging matters and has proposed a more coordinated and comprehensive plan to deal with the challenging issues of Singapore's aging population in the 21st century.

Funding Principles

Achieving coordinated and comprehensive planning of long-term care in Singapore requires that a number of key features of other health and social policy areas also be applied to this field. Thus, the principle of co-payment is being applied in long-term care as far as possible, as it applies in health and social services for the general population. The individual consumer and his or her family are expected to pay a portion of the charges while the government subsidizes the rest. This principle applies to the Medisave scheme, which is a compulsory medical savings scheme under the umbrella of the CPF. Medisave also demonstrates the second principle, that responsibility lies with the family unit, as savings can be used to meet the cost of parents' hospitalisation as well as for the individual's own expenses.

Third, access to publicly funded health and community care services for the elderly, such as home nursing, day care, and rehabilitation, is restricted by a variety of eligibility tests. A sliding scale of charges based on household income is imposed for these services, and only recipients of Public Assistance are entitled to free medical service at the government polyclinics. All other Singaporeans above age 60 are, however, entitled to a subsidy of 50% of the fees charged at these polyclinics. This principle of a sliding scale of means-tested fees will be refined and extended to long-term care services in the future.

FINANCIAL SECURITY AND COSTS OF CARE

A number of surveys of senior citizens in Singapore have found that most of the elderly are in favor of raising the retirement age from 55 years (Ministry of Social Affairs, 1983). The main reasons reported for not continuing to work were polarized: either sufficiency in financial support or ill health. Financial problems and boredom are cited as major difficulties during retirement (Government of Singapore, 1996). In the 1995 survey, only some 2% of seniors reported that their incomes were usually inadequate for their expenses. Among this small number, the most common reason stated was the high cost of living (58%).

Affordability of Health Care

A sizeable proportion of this group, close to 20%, reported experiencing high medical costs, and about half as many indicated that high medical costs were one of the factors contributing to feelings of financial insecurity for the future. Prolonging the period of employment could not only alleviate some of these problems; it could also maximize the productive capacity and capitalize on the experiences of older workers. Not only would it enable financial and social independence and provide the economic means to lead an active, healthy life in the community, but equally importantly, the period over which contributions could be made to the CPF and Medisave would be extended. As improvements in life expectancy continue, there will be a greater need to raise the age of retirement and to extend the working life of the older population. Various forms of incentives must be devised to encourage employers to retain older workers in active employment for as long as possible.

Over the last 15 years, the retirement age has been gradually raised in the public sector in Singapore. As an inducement to encourage more employers to retain older workers in their workforce, the employers' share of the contribution to the CPF for workers over the age of 55 has been substantially reduced. Actual workforce participation rate for the 55-60 age group for men and women has been gradually growing, especially for part-time work.

In Asia, only the more developed countries have public programs set up for the expressed objective of providing financial security in old age or, in cases of permanent disability, among the working population. As most of these schemes are relatively recent, the schemes will come into effect only when workers who have contributed to the savings schemes for many years retire. Although Singapore established its CPF almost 50 years ago, it has been estimated that, of those reaching age 60 in 2000, one in five men and one in three women have no CPF coverage, while about one in four of those who are covered will not have a balance sufficient to provide an adequate retirement income (Lee, 1999). Further, there are still sections of the workforce that are not covered by these formal systems, and these include the self-employed, family employers, casual workers, and others who work outside of permanent employment. Depending on the extent of savings or private insurance coverage among this group of workers, they are likely to lack financial security, posing problems in the future (Advisory Council on the Aged, 1989).

The present generation of the elderly lacks the financial security that will be available to younger cohorts with more substantial CPF savings and this has implications for financing both health and long-term care. Thus, their degree of financial dependency will continue to be high in the foreseeable future, and the present generation of the employed will have to bear the increasing costs of support for this group of elderly without personal savings, at the same time as saving for their own old age.

Although the health status of older Singaporeans is generally improving, the increased use of health care services among the aging population is already evident. In the *National Survey of Senior Citizens 1995* (Government of Singapore, 1996), about 7% of seniors aged 55 and over reported that they had been hospitalized within the past year, and this percentage increased with age, from 6% among those in the 55-64 age group, to 8% among those aged 65-74, and to 9% among those 75 years and above. Nearly 30% of seniors also indicated that they had been receiving regular treatment from doctors for some long-standing illness such as high blood pressure (52%), diabetes (32%), heart conditions (17%), rheumatism and arthritic conditions (11%), and stroke (3%).

Those aged 65 and over made up 7% of the population but accounted for 17% of all hospital admissions and 19% of outpatient polyclinic visits in 1995. Their average length of hospitalization was 11.3 days, substantially higher than the average for the overall population of about five days. The elderly consume a disproportionate share of health care due to increased prevalence of diseases that are chronic and more severe. Such demographic and epidemiological demand factors will exert economic pressures that are also likely to be aggravated by supply factors, such as the introduction of costly medical technologies.

INTEGRATING HEALTH CARE AND LONG-TERM CARE FINANCING

The Committee on the Problems of the Aged, convened in 1983, recommended measures to prevent, ameliorate, or deal with such problems, and its report set out a national policy covering aspects of employment, financial security, health and recreational needs, social services, institutional care, and family relations (Ministry of Health, 1984). Measures implemented at that time were reinforced by the Report of the Advisory Council on the Aged in 1989, which recommended the development of community-based programs for maintenance of good health, prevention of disease, rehabilitation, and social support for the elderly (Advisory Council on the Aged, 1989).

These measures were implemented in a manner consistent with the National Health Plan and the Medisave scheme, which in turn recognised that savings through the CPF were to form the backbone of viable financing of increasingly expensive health care for the elderly in Singapore over the longer term. Singapore has thus approached the financing of cost-effective health care for an expanding elderly population and implemented more sustainable methods of financing care within the framework of its overall old age security system. The official policy of enlarging the scope of mandatory savings to cover other areas is consistent with the social objectives of providing old age security. Since health care needs and expenses are expected to rise dramatically with aging, mechanisms to protect the elderly against expected medical costs were the first additions built into the CPF scheme.

In the Singapore context, financing health care through "pay-as-you-go" taxation or out of pocket payments would be inadequate to pay for high-quality health care, and prior savings, therefore, had to be enforced to meet the anticipated rising costs of medical care. These considerations formed the underlying basis for the National Health Plan of Singapore formulated in 1983. The key financing proposal of this plan, the Medisave scheme, imposed compulsory savings and restructured the existing system of medical care financing. The main objectives of the National Health Plan have been (1) to secure a healthy, fit, and productive population through active prevention and promotion of healthy lifestyles, and (2) to improve cost-efficiency in the health services. In addition to promoting individual responsibility for maintaining good health, the Plan has built up financial resources in order to create the means to pay for medical care during illness, especially in old age.

The 3-M Scheme

Savings for health care are based on the 3-M scheme of Medisave, Medishield, and Medifund.

- *Medisave* is the compulsory medical savings scheme linked to CPF accounts, and all employed people must contribute to a Medisave account up to the age of 55, with a minimum sum to be retained for health care in old age. Medisave accounts can also be pooled to pay for medical expenses of aged parents and grandparents who do not have their own accounts.
- *Medishield* is a supplementary back-up to Medisave that provides catastrophic illness insurance with premiums payable from Medisave accounts. It has a voluntary opt-out feature for those who have other health insurance coverage or who cannot afford the premiums.
- *Medifund* is an endowment fund for the poor and indigent who are without family support or do not have adequate Medisave or Medishield coverage. The fund is built up during periods of high economic growth to relieve the dependency on pay-as-you-go taxation as the primary means of financing social welfare for the poor (Phua, 1997).

The 3-M financing system covers expensive hospitalization and limited outpatient procedures, including selected non-acute care in community hospitals, which provide post-acute and rehabilitative care, and hospices. At present, most types of long-term care are excluded. Medisave withdrawals are limited to a maximum of $300 per day of hospital stay and according to the type of operations performed. These ceilings have not been adjusted despite several revisions in hospital fees. Due to the fixed limits, increasingly larger amounts of expenses for medical care are paid out-of-pocket.

There is voluntary opting-out in the Medishield scheme. This allows an element of choice for those who may have alternative coverage or those who may not be able to afford premiums that are risk-rated according to age. This is regressive to the older age groups, but the poor elderly who are uninsured for catastrophic illnesses can still fall back on the Medifund as a last resort. A Cost Review Committee in 1996 was concerned that one in four older Singaporeans over age 60 had opted out of the scheme. As this group is more likely to require health care, the Cost Review Committee noted that such a high rate of opting-out was undesirable.

Adequacy of Coverage for the Elderly

The current system of subsidies provides access to affordable health care for the elderly in the lower- and middle-income groups. In public hospitals, the subsidies range from 20% to 80% of the fees charged, depending on the ward class. In the government polyclinics, elderly patients pay only nominal fees with about 75% subsidy. It is expected that future generations of the elderly population will have built up enough Medisave savings and that the majority who will also have Medishield coverage will have sufficient financial resources to meet the cost of acute care. Those without adequate Medisave funds, Medishield coverage, or family support will rely on Medifund and other forms of financial assistance or charity.

Medisave can be used to pay for the hospital expenses of immediate family members, in line with the concept that the basic social and economic unit of the society is the family, and that caring for the welfare of ill and aged members of society is to remain first and foremost, a family responsibility. The aim is to preserve certain desirable values such as filial piety, and thereby serve to enhance the stability of an essential societal structure amidst rapid changes. Only when there are genuine difficulties, such as an entire family being unable to meet the medical expenses of its sick and elderly, are the costs subsidized from public taxes (Phua, 1986).

The 1995 National Survey in Singapore shows that Medisave has become the most important provision relied on by seniors aged 55 and above to finance their health care. More than half (55%) depended on their children's Medisave to pay for their medical expenses, while 18% depended on their own Medisave, and 2% on their spouse's Medisave. Medisave funds accounted for nearly 75% of the health care financing provisions of seniors, with the older groups relying on their children's Medisave more than their own. Further, two thirds of older women depended on their children's Medisave compared to 44% of men. As men were likely to have accumulated more in their Medisave accounts over their working lives, 30% of men were self-reliant for financing their health care, but only 7% of women. Approximately 10% of seniors had made no financial provisions for health care, either because unemployment or low income limited the capacity to accumulate Medisave or personal savings, or because they believed they could rely on their children to pay their medical bills if required.

One problem of the three-tiered approach is that some segments of the population who are currently not covered by the Medisave and Medishield schemes may not qualify for Medifund, which has very stringent eligibility conditions. These individuals must depend on other forms of financial assistance, mainly from their families.

To date, Singapore has sought to balance supply and demand in the health sector by deliberate manpower and facilities planning, and by mobilizing individual savings through the Medisave scheme within the CPF. Demand has been rationed implicitly through constraining consumer purchasing power in the market; the need for such constraint is all the more pressing since expectations of higher quality of services have risen with growing affluence (Phua, 1987).

FINANCING LONG-TERM CARE

There is presently no comprehensive system for financing long-term care in Singapore, and financing currently draws on five sources:

1. *Direct Payments* from older individuals and their families.
2. *Community Assistance* to voluntary welfare organizations, which secure up to 50% or more of their recurrent expenditure from fund raising.
3. *Government Funding* through grants-in-aid to VWOs, providing up to 90% of capital funding and up to 50% of recurrent funding, based on government cost norms, and 75% for Public Assistance cases.
4. *Extensions to Medisave* to provide limited coverage for selected forms of non-acute care as noted above.
5. Private operators are not present in greater numbers in long-term care due to the lack of financial incentives and problems in obtaining suitable premises due to prohibitive land and rental costs; there are also difficulties in recruiting staff as well as high labor costs for specialized and trained personnel.

To retain higher profits, private nursing homes either cater to the very rich by charging high fees for superior facilities or provide very basic or poor quality care to those with lower incomes. While the norm is to keep elderly family members in their own homes as long as possible, a number of problems have become evident in recent years. Although there is little statistical information on the types and quality of informal care provided to the elderly in their own homes, it is conceivable that most of the care is rendered by untrained relatives and maids. Lower-income families who cannot afford household help would be hard-pressed to provide good quality care to their elderly members. The increasing costs of care, without access to subsidies except for those receiving Public Assistance, could also create pressures on middle-income families, and the all-or-nothing situation with regard to access to subsidized nursing home care has only recently been addressed with the introduction of means testing that gives those with some income access to partial subsidies rather than none.

Due to the lack of long-term care alternatives and the limited financial assistance available, there can be perverse incentives to hospitalize since the current 3-M financing system covers only hospitalization. The present hospital subsidy system may also explain the longer lengths of stay in the lower-class wards, since lower-income patients and their working class families cannot afford the direct or indirect costs of alternative care at home. Since subsidies for home medical care and home nursing care are limited to the poor and indigent, currently perverse incentives exist to admit elderly to nursing homes when they could possibly be served more cost-effectively in their own homes.

The present bias in funding to nursing homes is likely to increase, not so much due to policy promotion of this form of care but because of cost pressures underlying even controlled expansion of nursing homes. Capital grants to VWO homes increased by 18% from 1998 to 1999, when the total of S$53.5m was divided between $22.5m for capital projects and $31m for operating expenditure (Yong, 2000). These capital grants carry future commitments to operating costs that will have to be met by a mix of government funding, increased fund raising, and increased fees. Notwithstanding the commitment to support families in providing care for their elderly, there has been no comprehensive funding for community care services and long-term care in the recent past.

RECENT INITIATIVES AND FUTURE OPTIONS

Based on recommendations of the IMC, several recent initiatives have been taken in Singapore that extend provisions for long-term care within the wider framework of the CPF and the 3-M scheme, and that maintain the role of government as a partner with families and VWOs.

Diversifying Funding Sources

Two initiatives were taken in early 2000. First, an Elder Care Fund was set up under the Medical and Elderly Care Endowment Schemes Act to finance the future operating subsidies of VWOs. Initial capital injections of $500m through 2000 are to be built up to a target of $2.5 billion by 2010. Second, means testing has been introduced in VWO nursing homes with a sliding scale of subsidies from 25% to 75%, taking account of household size and income. Prior to this, other forms of community care have not been means-tested, in contrast to the medical and health services, which provide discounts for elderly patients or waivers for those on Public Assistance.

More indirectly, a Community Health Screening program, "Check Your Health," has been introduced with a view to limiting future costs of long-term care. The program focuses on detecting diabetes, high blood pressure, and high cholesterol among those aged 55 and over. The three-year program is expected to cost $6.5m.

A second round of initiatives was announced in January 2001, when a number of recommendations made by the IMC, through the Working Group on Health Care, were endorsed by the government. Principal among these is the move to restructure funding of VWOs in a way that provides incentives for them to raise more funds and to cover an increased volume of patients, including more fee paying clients, and to improve the quality of care quite substantially in order to attract the higher income. Under the previous arrangements, grants to VWOs were capped or reduced once the VWO raised excess funds. These arrangements not only provided little incentive to raise funds, but they could, in fact, penalise VWOs that did raise additional funds.

At present, government funding for 90% of capital costs does not differentiate between the types of residential care, such as quality of amenities and level of comfort in the physical environment. The recommendation to fund on a "cost-per-bed" basis also does not take into consideration special requirements and needs of different services to be provided. Government funding for recurrent costs also does not differentiate specifically the case-mix of patients, like age, gender, severity of disease, and complicated conditions. It may be desirable to target the limited government subsidies to those in greatest need and have more refined subventions to balance the affordability of patients and their families with means-tested user charges.

Further Savings and Insurance Options

Beyond the initiatives that recently have been supported by the government, the IMC recommended the establishment of additional financing for long-term care, called "Step-Down Care." The proposals included an insurance scheme to help individuals and their families defray the high costs of step-down care required by those elderly with very severe functional disabilities. The IMC concluded that the best option for financing would be along the lines of the Medishield scheme. Like the Medishield scheme, a Long-Term Care Insurance (LTCI) Scheme would be voluntary, based on an opting out approach, and have the features of deductibles and co-insurance to discourage over-consumption and over-servicing. There is concern that the number and proportion of those who have opted out of Medishield could be repeated in any long-term care insurance scheme established on a voluntary basis. Of greater concern is the large number of young people who have opted out of Medishield, despite the relatively cheaper premiums that are already adjusted to their lower risk-ratings. It will become increasingly unfair for those remaining in the smaller pool to have to bear the burden of carrying the risks of the elderly, especially if those who have opted out and have not contributed earlier are allowed to opt in later without any penalties.

The costs of such a scheme under varying assumptions have been analysed by Valdez, Tan, and Wong (2000), who recommend augmenting the CPF by way of adding a separate and compulsory Medisave account for long-term care. The advantages of this approach are noted as the capacity to base contribution rates on sound actuarial calculations and so ensure financial stability, minimization of administrative costs, and mandatory enrollment that avoids the market failures of moral hazard and adverse selection. A pre-funded scheme providing partial cover is also seen as enabling control of the costs of long-term care in the future. The authors note, however, that while LTCI could provide a solution for the future generations of Singapore's elderly, a pre-funded scheme will not finance the long-term care needs of the current elderly generation.

Recent policy announcements have promised more government matching grants-in-aid for VWOs to work with grassroots organizations through the Community Development Councils. Many of these new funding mechanisms are directed at the local government infrastructure development to cater to the needs of aging constituents. The deliberations of the IMC have focused public attention on the financing issues concerning the provision of long-term care. Other recommendations included a review of capital funding for VWOs to build step-down care facilities, a means test to channel government subsidy for step-down care to those patients most in need of financial help, and government subsidies to support home medical care and home nursing services. The details of the financing proposals for these measures are still being scrutinized and evaluated because they have major financial implications for the government.

Singapore's policy and financing arrangements for income security, health care and long-term care exemplify what the World Bank has termed the "pillars" approach to meeting the costs of population aging through a mix of systems: taxation, savings, and insurance. These pillars have, however, taken a different form in Singapore than in most other countries. Building on a clearly recognized base of family financial support and care for the elderly, the main financing pillar is individual savings organised through the government-mandated CPF and Medisave. The role of the government-funded pillars of Medifund and the new ElderCare Fund are built on taxation and are targeted at the poor by strict eligibility criteria and means testing. The planned LTCI scheme would build a further pillar for the future, but again, based on individual savings, with some degree of cost sharing and risk pooling. It is expected that this mix of financing systems based on the savings approach would be more sustainable for supporting the basic functions of Singapore's system of old age security, and avoid the intergenerational transfers inherent in pay-as-you-go financing through conventional taxation or social insurance.

REFERENCES

Advisory Council on the Aged (1989). *Report of the Advisory Council on the Aged.* Ministry of Community Development, Singapore.

Government of Singapore (1996). *The National Survey of Senior Citizens in Singapore 1995.* Ministry of Health, Ministry of Community Development, Ministry of Labour, Department of Statistics, Ministry of Trade & Industry, and the National Council of Social Services, November 1996.

Lee, W. K. M. (1999). Economic and social implications of aging in Singapore. *Journal of Aging & Social Policy, 10*(4): 73-92.

Ministry of Community Development (1999). *Report of the Inter-Ministerial Committee on the Ageing Population.* Ministry of Community Development, Singapore.

Ministry of Health (1999). *Report of the Inter-Ministerial Committee on Health Care for the Elderly,* Ministry of Health, Singapore.

Ministry of Health (1984). *Report of the Committee on the Problems of the Aged.* Ministry of Health, Singapore.

Ministry of Social Affairs (1983). *Report on the National Survey of Senior Citizens.* Ministry of Social Affairs, Singapore.

Phillips, D. R. (1992). *Ageing in East and South-East Asia.* London: Edward Arnold.

Phua, K. H. (1986). Singapore's family savings scheme. *World Health,* May 1986.

Phua, K. H. (1987). Saving for Health. *World Health Forum, 8:* 38-41.

Phua, K. H. (1987). Ageing: Socio-economic implications for health care in Singapore. *Annals Academy of Medicine, 16*(1): 15-23.

Phua, K. H., Seow, A., & Lee, H. P. (1996). Issues and challenges of public health in the 21st Century in Singapore, in Khairuddin, Y., Low, Y. L., & Zulkifli, S. N.

(Eds.), *Issues and Challenges of Public Health in the 21st Century*. Kuala Lumpur: University of Malaya Press.

Phua, K. H. (1997). Medical savings accounts and health care financing in Singapore, in Schieber, G. (Ed.), *Innovations in Health Care Financing*. World Bank Discussion Paper No. 365: 247-255.

Phua, K. H., & Yap, M. T. (1998). Financing health care–Singapore Case Study, in Prescott, N. (Ed.), *Choices in Financing Health Care and Old Age Security*. World Bank Discussion Paper No. 392.

Shantakumar, G. (1994). *The Aged Population of Singapore*. Census of Population 1990, Monograph No. 1, Singapore.

Sherraden, M. (1970). Provident funds and social protection: The case of Singapore, in Midgley, J. & Sherraden, M. (Eds.), *Alternatives to Social Security: An International Inquiry*. Westport, CT: Auburn House.

Siegel, J. S., & Hoover, S. L. (1982). Demographic aspects of health of the elderly to the year 2000 and beyond. *World Health Statistics Quarterly*, *35*(3/4): 140-1.

United Nations (1991). *Population Ageing in Asia*, Asian Population Studies Series No. 108. Economic and Social Commission for Asia and the Pacific (ESCAP), Bangkok, and Japanese Organization for International Cooperation in Family Planning Inc., Tokyo.

Valdez, E. A., Tan, K. C., & Wong, Y. W. (2000). Funding long-term care in Singapore. *Hallym International Journal of Ageing*, *2*(1): 70-84.

World Bank (1994). *Averting the Old Age Crisis: Policies to Protect the Old and Promote Growth*. New York: Oxford University Press.

World Health Organization (1999). *Ageing and Health: A Global Challenge for the 21st Century*, WHO Centre for Health Development, Kobe, Japan.

Yong, L. S. (2000). *Country Report on Health and Aging, Singapore*. Paper presented at WHO Workshop on Health and Aging: Research, Education, Policy and Practice, Adelaide, Australia.

Organization and Delivery of Long-Term Care in Singapore: Present Issues and Future Challenges

Kalyani K. Mehta, PhD
S. Vasoo, PhD

National University of Singapore

SUMMARY. This paper focuses on the Singaporean model of long-term care for older people. With only about 2% of the older population living in institutions, the mainstay of long-term care is community care. The reader is provided an overview of the Singaporean services, including case management, followed by a discussion of the current issues

Dr. Kalyani K. Mehta is Associate Professor, Department of Social Work and Psychology, National University of Singapore. She has done research on elderly services and policies for the past 10 years, has published articles in international and regional journals, and presented conference papers in the United States, China, Australia, and South East Asia. As a member of the National Committee on the Aged as well as a consultant to the United Nations Economic and Social Commission for Asia and the Pacific (ESCAP), Dr. Mehta has recommended policies and services for the improved quality of life of older persons. Her edited volume, *Untapped Resources: Women in Aging Societies Across Asia* (1997), added greatly to the literature on the status and roles of older women in aging societies. Her research interests include family caregiving, religion and aging, widowhood, remarriage, and cross-cultural patterns of aging.

Dr. S. Vasoo is Associate Professor, Department of Social Work and Psychology, National University of Singapore. He is actively involved as an advisor to many social and community organizations, including NGOs of senior citizens. He is a member of the Inter-Ministerial Committee on Ageing and has chaired its Committee on Social Integration of the Elderly. He studies voluntary action of the elderly.

Both authors can be contacted at the National University of Singapore, 10 Kent Ridge Crescent, Singapore 119260 (Dr. Kalyani Mehta's E-mail: swkkkm@nus.edu.sg; Dr. S. Vasoo's E-mail: swkvasoo@nus.edu.sg).

[Haworth co-indexing entry note]: "Organization and Delivery of Long-Term Care in Singapore: Present Issues and Future Challenges." Mehta, Kalyani K., and S. Vasoo. Co-published simultaneously in *Journal of Aging & Social Policy* (The Haworth Press, Inc.) Vol. 13, No. 2/3, 2001, pp. 185-201; and: *Long-Term Care in the 21st Century: Perspectives from Around the Asia-Pacific Rim* (ed: Iris Chi, Kalyani K. Mehta, and Anna L. Howe) The Haworth Press, Inc., 2001, pp. 185-201. Single or multiple copies of this article are available for a fee from The Haworth Document Delivery Service [1-800-HAWORTH, 9:00 a.m. - 5:00 p.m. (EST). E-mail address: getinfo@haworthpressinc.com].

and future challenges. In keeping with the prospect of a rapidly aging population profile, the Singapore government plays a leading role in framing policy and planning for future needs of this sector of the population.

KEYWORDS. Aging policy, long-term care, Singapore

THE NEED FOR CARE

The demographic revolution of population aging that was well advanced in most developed countries by the end of the 20th century is evident in Asia, too. After Japan, Singapore is the fastest aging nation in the Asia Pacific region, and in recognition of the significance of this development, an Inter-Ministerial Committee (IMC) on Health Care and another on the Aging Population were convened by the Singapore Government in 1997 and 1998, respectively. The IMCs released two reports on their deliberations in 1999, and these reports both review the need for care and preview the challenges that are likely to be forthcoming in the early years of the 21st century.

As an island state with a total resident population of just over 3.5 million in 2000, the impact of the demographic processes of population aging is highly visible in Singapore. Life expectancy at birth is already high, at 75 years for males and nearly 80 years for females, and these figures are expected to rise further. The demographic data given in Table 1 show that the proportion of the population aged 65 and over will almost double from 7.3% in 1999 to 13.1% in 2020, and by 2030, close to one in every five Singaporeans will be aged 65 and over. Within this rapidly aging demographic profile, the increase of those in late life, above 75 years, is even more conspicuous.

The doubling of the proportion aged 65 and over in Singapore will occur in a far shorter time, less than 25 years, compared to up to 150 years in the already older countries of western Europe, and around 80 years in the developed Pacific Rim countries of North America, Australia, and New Zealand, which are now reaching the 14% mark (ESCAP, 1996). The speed of this demographic transition has major implications not only for health and social services but for other sectors of society as well, and the planning of long-term care for the elderly population requires consideration of both the development of formal services and the changing roles of families in informal care.

TABLE 1. Characteristics of Aged Population, Singapore, 1999-2030

Characteristic	1999	2000	2020	2030
Aged 65+ ('000)	235	312	529	796
Proportion of total population aged 65 and over	7.3	8.4	13.1	18.9
Median Age (Yrs)	33.4	36.9	39.3	41.2
Dependency Ratio Total	42.0	38.7	44.9	56.4
Young (0-14 years)	31.7	27.1	25.9	26.9
Old (65+ years)	10.4	11.6	19.0	29.5

Source: Singapore Department of Statistics, cited in the Inter-Ministerial Report, 1999: 29

Changing Family Structures and Roles

The IMC has noted that one key concern is that the sheer rise in the numbers and proportion of older persons could potentially put stress on families and eldercare services (IMC Report, 1999b). As in other Asian countries, the family in Singapore has been providing the major part of care and support for elderly family members (Knodel & Debavalya, 1997). Although there are no strong data to show that families are shirking their filial responsibilities, several social and demographic changes mitigate against the continuity of family care as the primary form of eldercare in Singapore.

These trends take on added importance in the context of the present paradigm of eldercare in Singapore, which is a partnership among the government, the community, and the family (Mehta, 2000). In tandem with the "Many Helping Hands" policy of the Ministry of Community Development, the community and the government are expected to lend a hand to aging families in order to reduce the stress of caregiving for older members. Reiterating the government's long-standing position at the opening of a conference on choices in financing health care and old age security, convened under the auspices of the World Bank in Singapore in 1997, the Minister for Health noted that "the family setting is still the best approach; it provides the elderly with the warmth and companionship of family members and a level of emotional support which cannot be found elsewhere" (Prescott, 1998).

In line with this partnership approach, the government encourages voluntary welfare organizations (VWOs) in their efforts to offer quality long-term care in the community through provision of financial and other forms of support. These services and programs are discussed in detail below, but it is becoming apparent to many in government, in VWOs, and in the community at large that with rising numbers of older Singaporeans, non-family partners will be required to play bigger roles over the next few decades.

Declining mortality and low fertility rates mean that the aged are being recognized as a more integral part of Singaporean society. As in Japan, the Singapore government recognizes that a large proportion of citizens is fast approaching the age of retirement, and acknowledges the implications of aging for policy-making and government expenditures. There is a concern to maintain the health and vitality of the elderly as their life spans increase, so that the older population does not become an unduly heavy financial and social burden on the society. Perhaps even more so than in Japan, the Singapore government sees a viable family structure that is able to provide love, care, and support for its elderly members as crucial, and indeed the ideal, if the formal support system for the elderly is to be kept to a minimum.

At the same time, and notwithstanding a continuing Confucian value system, the traditional caregivers of the family, and more specifically female relatives, are coming under increasing pressures from modernization and urbanization. These changes include a shift to dual-income nuclear families, living apart from older generations, increasing levels of education and high rates of participation in the formal workforce for women, more young Singaporeans working and living abroad, more single elderly among the generation for whom family formation was interrupted by World War II, and changing social values. Two demographic indicators point to the extent of these intergenerational changes.

First, age-specific sex ratios provide an indicator of need for health care services arising from the interaction of advancing age, gender differences in chronic diseases, and social support from spouses. In the 1990 census, men constituted 47% of the aged population, but the sex ratio dropped from 97 males per 100 females at age 60 to 69 years, to 80 in the 70-79 age group, and only 60 at 80 years and above. Since women generally outlive men and mortality rates are falling faster among females than males, the net result is a growing sex imbalance, especially with increasing age (Shantakumar 1994, 1995). The health problems of the elderly consequently reflect the conditions and needs of a larger proportion of older women, and as women generally use health services more often than men, differential demand will be increasingly pronounced in future. The lower sex ratio with increasing age does not of itself necessarily lead to a higher demand for social services, as family structure and marital status come into play. Again in the 1990 census, 29% of the aged population were widowed, but the figure was 54% for aged women compared to about 19% for aged men.

Second, the ratio of the elderly to the working-age population, the old age dependency ratio, is projected to increase from around 10 currently to 30 by 2030. The need for more old people to be supported by a proportionately smaller working population has major implications for labor supply and financial security, and for the provision of social services, especially health care, as alternatives or adjuncts to family care (Teo, 1994). Population movements due to changes in living arrangements and employment patterns can exacerbate the need for external assistance (Ministry of Health, 1984).

Vulnerable Groups

Given the differentials in aging patterns, not all older persons require continual care. However, those in the "old old" and "very old" categories are generally more likely to need constant supervision, social and emotional support as well as instrumental help. Focusing on these categories as the potential target groups for care services, population projections show that the 75-and-over age group will increase even faster than the 60-75 years age group (Cheung, 1993). This older group is at risk of needing care and attention, and as more family resources will have to be drawn into attending to the social and physical requirements of very old relatives, some families are likely to face considerable stress in providing care to the sick and disabled.

Another vulnerable category are aged couples living on their own, who have increased from 9% of households with persons aged 60 years and above in 1990 to 15% in 1997. Poor older people living alone are also identified as being at risk, and the aging process has become especially apparent in housing estates that were constructed in the 1960s. There are increasing numbers of older senior citizens living in these estates, and it is urgent that community groups and organizations begin to plan the establishment of more community-based programs such as day care, meals programs, home-help service and domiciliary nursing care, and crisis-response services. In taking a proactive approach to initiate a network of services in older housing estates, it will be possible to provide support for families with vulnerable aged relatives and minimize disruptions to the social and economic lives of the families.

SERVICES PROVIDED BY THE SOCIAL WELFARE SYSTEM

Those involved in developing community-based services in Singapore can draw on several decades of experience in the United Kingdom and in the United States and other countries that have sought to expand community care as an alternative to institutional care (Challis & Davies, 1986; Gordon & Donald, 1993). As well as recognising that the trend towards community-based long-term care is not only feasible but also the preferred choice of the elderly themselves, as in other countries, Singapore is starting from a very different position. With only some 2% of its elderly living in institutions at present, Singapore is well-placed to embark on the development of community care as the mainstay of long-term care rather than as an alternative to the kind of large, long-established, and costly institutional care sectors that most other countries are seeking to counter.

The paradigm of elder care in Singapore has been evolving for some time now and as with other areas of health and social services, a distinctive Singapore model has emerged. Three main features of this model are the interweaving of informal and formal care to suit the needs of individual clients and their families; the support of a diversity of VWOs to provide a range of services and develop innovative projects in service delivery, including case management; and the attention given to improving health and well-being among vulnerable groups with a view to reducing future needs for long-term care services. The range of services now available is summarized in Table 2, which shows the different levels of care provided by sub-systems of home-based, community-based, and residential services. The following account focuses on community care, detailing the non-institutional services delivered to the home and semi-institutional services based in the community.

Who Are the Providers of Community-Based Long-Term Care?

The main providers are voluntary welfare organisations (VWOs), with the private sector playing a role only in the delivery of nursing home care. As of January 2000, there were 24 private sector nursing homes compared to VWO provision of 23 nursing homes, three hospices, and one residential facility for dementia patients. In addition, there were four community hospitals and two hospitals for the chronically sick.

The Ministry of Community Development and Sports and the Ministry of Health support the efforts of VWOs and administer mechanisms for quality management. As well as mandatory guidelines for nursing homes, the Ministry of Community Development and Sports has issued a set of guidelines for community-based services for the elderly. The guidelines are strongly recommended but not mandatory (Ministry of Community Development, 1998). A third statutory body, the National Council of Social Service, plays a coordinating role among non-government welfare organizations and helps in representing their views to the government.

TABLE 2. Long-Term Care Services and Programs in Singapore

Community care		Institutional care
Home-based (non-institutional)	**Community-based (semi-institutional)**	**Residential services**
1. Socio-recreational 2. Befriending/counselling 3. "Doorstep" services delivered in the home	1. Day activity centres 2. Social Centres 3. Day Care Centres and Rehabilitation Centres	1. Sheltered homes 2. Hospices 3. Nursing Homes (private & VWOs) 4. Community Hospitals

Day Care and Home Modification Services

In 1998, there were 20 day care and rehabilitation centers distributed across the island and operated by a variety of government and non-government organizations. Six are Senior Citizens' Health Care Centres that offer both social and health care programs especially for patients newly discharged from acute hospitals. These services play a crucial role in the smooth transition of elderly from acute care to home care. Family caregivers are given informal training at these centers. Three day care centers specialize in the care of elderly suffering from dementia.

Other day centers are operated by secular and religious organizations, for example, the Wan Qing Lodge and the Adventist Church. Some day centers are located within the premises of residential homes, thus providing a dual function for the latter as well as a source of income generation. Day care centers have been found to help relieve the stress of family caregivers by providing respite care and ensuring the safety of the elderly, especially if other family members are not at home during the day (Kua, 1987).

In planning to meet the projected increase in need for day care centers, there has been some experimentation in different forms of provision. One such experiment takes the form of 3-in-1 centers, where day care for three age groups is located within one vicinity. Bringing young children, school-age children, and elderly together in intergenerational programs such as the celebration of festivals, teaching of handicrafts, and community singing inculcates a greater sense of affiliation between the generations.

There are 11 social day centers that cater mainly to the relational and social needs of elderly citizens. These centers are neighborhood hubs characterized by informality and self-management by the senior citizens. Most are located within Family Service Centres and require minimal funds and manpower because volunteers, including robust young elderly, are the backbone of these programs.

Day activity centers are different again in that they meet the needs of low-income elderly who live alone in government flats. This vulnerable group has been identified as needing community support and companionship, and the day activity centers are linked to a joint project between the Ministry of Community Development and the Housing Development Board (HDB), the statutory body in charge of the government-housing program. A reputable voluntary welfare organization is selected by the Ministry to run the day activity centers with a lean staff and a large volunteer input. The day activity center provides an opportunity for social interaction for these poor and lonely elderly and a contact to depend on in times of crisis. Together, the day care and rehabilitation centers offer comprehensive services for the senior citizens living with their family members, while the day activity centers offer social and emergency services for the poor elderly living alone.

A further function of the HDB is the upgrading of the low-rent, one-room flats at no cost to tenants. Installation of elderly-friendly amenities, such as non-slip tiles in the bathroom, handle bars, and pedestal toilets, and an alarm system that alerts neighbors and the day activity center nearby of an emergency, are the main features of this Congregate Housing project that in the last seven years has been expanded to 25 blocks, each housing approximately 150 elder tenants.

Home Care Services

Care services delivered in the home, or "door-step" programs as they are known in Singapore, provide a wide range of services for vulnerable and frail older people, including home help and household chores, meal delivery, escort to polyclinics and hospitals, home nursing and home medical care, and befriending services. The organizations concerned usually draw geographical boundaries for their services due to limited resources, both financial and manpower.

Other community-based services are located in the VWO rather than being delivered to the home. These include telephone hotlines for counseling, face-to-face casework and counseling, caregiver support groups, and weekly lunches prepared by volunteers. There are two key organizations, the Singapore Action Group of Elders (SAGE) and the Tsao Foundation, that specialize in the delivery of aged care services. The former not only provides direct services but also has a Centre for the Study of Ageing (CENSA) because research is seen to be of paramount importance in charting changing profiles and needs of successive cohorts of elderly in Singapore's fast-changing society. The

Tsao Foundation, in contrast, focuses on the delivery of medical services to low-income elderly and the training of informal caregivers; it also runs an Acupuncture clinic. Other voluntary bodies provide free Chinese medical treatment, in one case via a mobile clinic staffed by volunteer doctors.

Socio-Recreational Services

Socio-recreational community-based programs form an integral part of the repertoire of elderly services and are directed to the "young old" who are usually active and desire to remain productive members of society. The Retired and Senior Volunteer Program (RSVP) provides an avenue for professional and educated retired senior citizens. For the wider majority, there are almost 400 Senior Citizens' Clubs (SCC) established by the People's Association scattered across the island. Most SCCs are located in Community Centres, which are multi-purpose, secular centers catering to the general Singaporean population, regardless of age, ethnicity, or religion. Programs organized by the SCCs include tours to Malaysia, dancing, singing, exercise classes such as Tai Chi and Qigong, and competitions between clubs. The SCCs play a very active part in the celebrations for Senior Citizens' Week held in November every year.

Some of the social programs have an emphasis on education. For example, SAGE offers a program of lifelong learning that includes Chinese calligraphy and traditional crafts, and other organizations conduct training in computer skills, training for family caregivers, and enrichment skills. As future cohorts of Singaporean elderly will be better educated and will have greater savings, there is likely to be a greater demand for these programs.

Case Management

The introduction of case management in Singapore illustrates the way in which a distinctive Singaporean approach has been developed from the experience of other countries. Besides using case management to address the problems of duplication, fragmentation, and frustration for consumers as reported by Austin (1986) and Schneider et al. (2000) and to achieve added cost-effectiveness in comparison to institutionalization as argued by Greene et al. (1998), Singapore has embraced case management as a means to gaining wider benefits of community development (Atchley, 2000).

The National Council of Social Service (NCSS) launched a two-year pilot project in case management in May 1998 through the Tsao Foundation and SAGE. In this project, case management was defined as a new service that involves the assessment of an elderly person's health and psychological and social needs, and maximization of services to attain optimal and most cost-effective care of the elderly and their caregivers to prevent unnecessary institutionalization (SAGE, 1998). This strategy of service delivery is being examined to mitigate the problems of uneven distribution and fragmentation in service delivery, and aims to develop viable models of case management to suit the Singapore context.

Since public awareness of services is relatively low, as evident from the 1995 National Survey of Senior Citizens (Ministry of Health, 1996), and services are often dispersed and fragmented, the case management concept is attractive in Singapore's context. It is, however, a costly service, and the IMC has noted that case management needs to be closely targeted to those who need it most, namely the poorly-educated senior citizens without families or the frail senior citizens with multiple needs and problems (Ministry of Community Development, 1999b).

Eligibility criteria for the pilot project were frail elderly, 60 years and older, regardless of gender or ethnicity, who required three or more community-based services, and whose gross household income did not exceed S$2000 per month. The SAGE project covers applicants in the Central geographical region and the Tsao Foundation project covers the Western region. At present, the National Council of Social Service funded the project, including the salaries of the staff, but in time it may be expanded to higher income groups on a paid basis.

The SAGE Case Management Service offers more than 15 different types of services to a caseload of 76 clients, as of January 2000. The initial holistic assessment is very thorough, covering demographic, family, medical, financial, and psychosocial dimensions. Most referrals to date have come from a government hospital in the Central region, and other sources include family service centers and VWOs. The staff includes two professionals and one administrative support officer. A brokerage model is used, whereby no direct service is rendered but the case manager taps the community-based services and coordinates them for the client's benefit. During the two-year pilot period, the service has been provided free of charge to users.

The problems identified in this pilot project have been a shortage and lack of training of volunteers, pressure of time when services must be arranged prior to a client's discharge from hospital, monitoring of quality and efficiency of services, and lastly, difficulties in meeting ethnic preferences of diet of the clients, especially minority groups. Much time is spent building rapport with family members where they are involved since a family-oriented approach is applied.

While the case-management team at SAGE consists of social workers, the Tsao Foundation team consists of a psychologist and a retired nurse. This team is linked to a home medical team at the Tsao Foundation's Hua Mei Clinic, facilitating provision of immediate medical care and guidance where necessary. The SAGE team relies on doctors from the hospital of referral as well as nurses from the Home Nursing Foundation for medical support. At the end of the pilot project, the NCSS conducted an evaluation to determine the feasibility of continuation of the project. Positive outcomes were identified, thus leading to the expansion of the Case Management Service to three organizations altogether.

CURRENT ISSUES–FUTURE CHALLENGES

In the Singapore context, the mechanism of IMCs has proved to be highly effective. The Committee consists of high-level representatives from the ministries concerned, as well as other relevant statutory boards and selected voluntary welfare organizations. At the initial stage, the IMC is assigned the task of collating data as well as feedback from the public with regard to the matter at hand. At the later stage, when the report of the IMC is released, the status of the Committee can change into a standing Committee. The standing IMC is a national-level, policymaking and decision-taking tool established by the state to integrate policies and services in a particular sector or for a particular population. The IMC on Ageing Population currently oversees the implementation of the recommendations of the Report. Needed resources, such as funding and staff, are also channeled to the respective sector to ensure that the process is smooth and efficient. In multidisciplinary areas such as aging, where several ministries are involved, such a strategy is highly apt and effective. With the state's backing, the recommendations tend to be translated into reality with minimum barriers.

Through 1999, six working groups convened by the Inter-Ministerial Committee on the Aging Population provided the means for assessing the present status of Singapore's long-term care services and identifying the issues that will have to be addressed to meet future needs. The working groups have been effective in generating feedback from various sectors of the population, and the IMC has initiated the crafting of a national strategy to deal with the challenges of an aging society in the coming decades. The scope of the IMC illustrates that long-term care is viewed in the wider context of aging in Singapore.

As a standing committee of the government, the IMC oversees the implementation of the resulting recommendations. It also serves as a coordinating body between the relevant Ministries, thus enhancing the prospects for a system of integrated service delivery. In its 1999 report, the IMC put forward proposals for two major service innovations and made six other suggestions for consideration by policymakers. It was clear from the outset that the IMC would be a standing committee, tasked to "Steer and guide the comprehensive, holistic and coordinated development of policies and programs for the elderly; review such policies and programs periodically . . . " (*Straits Times*, 15/11/98).

Service Innovations

The first proposal for service innovation was the establishment of Multi-Service Centres across the island. These centers are conceptualized as centralized locations for the integration of health, social, and other community-based services. When implemented, they would contribute to boosting the array of services that are available but not easily accessible for the elderly and their families. The Multi-Service Centres would be at the core of the Five-Year Strategic Plan for an aging population. The government has announced its intention to allocate $(Singapore)30 million towards setting up three centers to be ready by 2005.

The second proposal is for Golden Manpower Centres (GMCs), which would work with the Ministry of Manpower Career Centres and provide information, training, job placement, and access to voluntary work for older workers and retired people, particularly those with less education. Low-income elderly tend to form the majority of older workers who are least likely to find jobs due to their low levels of education and lack of skills. If these GMCs can provide training as well as job placement, poverty and health deterioration could be prevented. Retirement age in Singapore is currently 62, but the labor participation rate of those between the ages 55-62 years is relatively low. In 1997, the labor force participation rate for older persons 55-64 years was only 43%, while in Japan it was 67%, and the GMCs are seen as having a role in keeping more older workers in the workforce.

Policy Issues

The first of the five policy issues identified by the IMC is how to contain the cost pressures associated with demands for setting up more and more institutional care programs. The pressures are largely coming from families seeking alternative care arrangements, as well as from hospitals wanting to discharge patients who no longer require acute care. In seeking a balance between institutional and community-based services, projections of future needs have been made by the IMC, as set out in Table 3. It is evident that community services are already lagging behind the planning ratios, especially in home nursing and home help. Substantial additional resources are needed to reach the targets set for community care services in the future, but these resources are still fewer than those required for institutional care even within the target levels. Unless strictly controlled, expansion of institutional services will place an even greater burden on the government, which in turn would lead to higher taxation on the public, and at the same time, undermine the development of community care.

The path that Singapore intends to take is to examine how more preventive and community-based programs can be organized and delivered effectively in an integrated manner. This approach is consistent with the overall national policy of encouraging active and successful aging. The community emphasis will make services accessible and enable aging-in-place for the elderly, with concomitant community mobilization. It is believed that such a strategy will make the programs more cost-effective and help the elderly and their families to remain independent.

The second policy issue concerns manpower for long-term care. The combination of a well-educated, highly skilled labor force and a high demand for labor in Singapore means that, along with many areas of economic activity, long-term care faces a shortage of trained nurses, occupational therapists, and physiotherapists. A large proportion of staff aides in residential care institutions already consists of foreign workers, giving rise to cultural and communication problems. Residential care facilities and day care centers must train these staff members in the areas of dialects, attitudes, and skills in working with older people, in particular the frail and terminally ill. Another area that is likely to demand more attention in future is the training of family caregivers and volunteers to increase their effectiveness.

Third, in canvassing the need for more innovative elderly services suited to the local context to further the development of community-based long-term care, the promotion of community care cooperatives has been seriously discussed. The National Trade Union Congress (NTUC) has embarked on its first Eldercare Cooperative. As conceived, these cooperatives would provide a range of services at affordable rates, including home help, meal service, transport and escort service, employment placement, and day care. Members of the cooperatives would be eligible for rebates if they choose to use the services. Community mobilization of retirees, housewives, and even students looking for part-time employment could provide the much-needed manpower. For transport, voluntary organizations and residents could form a transport pool to meet the needs of elderly who require transport and companionship for the purpose of follow-up medical treatment. A well-managed database could match needs of residents in the vicinity with organizations and suppliers of skills or equipment. The cooperatives can be viable because volunteers and some paid staff will manage them on a not-for-profit basis. The notion of the common ownership of the cooperative *by* the members and *for* the members will be the key to the success of such cooperatives. Other innovative ideas have

TABLE 3. Projected Need for Elderly Health Services, 2000 to 2030

Types of Services	Planning Ratio per 1000 aged 65 and over	Projection number of places needed				
		1997	2000	2010	2020	2030
Day Rehabilitation and Day Care Places*	3.5 places per 1,000	761 (701)	821 [820]	1,100	1,900	2,800
Home Medical Care	5 elderly needing 1 visit per month per 1,000	1,087 (750)	1,173 [825]	1,600	2,700	4,000
Home Nursing	15 elderly needing 2 visits per month per 1,000	6,522 (5,000)	7,035 [5,500]	9,400	15,900	24,000
Home Help	4 per 1000 needing daily visits	870 (255)	938 [300]	1,250	2,120	3,200
Acute Geriatric Beds	1 per 1000 elderly	217 (188)	235 [226]	310	530	800
Geriatric Specialist	1 per 10,000 elderly	22 (15)	25 [21]	30	55	80
Community Hospital Beds *	3.5 per 1000 elderly	761 (426)	820 [426]	1090	1855	2800
Chronic sick Beds *	1.5 per 1000 elderly	326 (218)	352 [218]	480	800	1200
Nursing Home Beds incl. for dementia patients *	28 beds per 1000	6087 (4703)	6566 [5635]	8800	14,900	22,400

Source: Report of the Inter-Ministerial Committee on Health-Care for Elderly, 1999
Notes: ( ) availability in 1997
    [ ] estimated availability in year 2000
    * Estimated availability will improve by the year 2003: Community Hospital Beds to 940, Chronic Sick Hospital Beds to 400 and Nursing Home Beds to 7300

been proposed to expand services such as telephone contact, community kitchens manned by ethnic self-help community organizations, and caregiver support groups, as well as elderly self-help groups.

The growth of service provision through involving community organizations is highly consistent with the government policy of encouraging affordable and accessible community-based services. A further important corollary of this approach is that services provided by community organizations do not carry the stigma that is often attached to usage of "voluntary welfare" services. The emphasis on self-help organizations is also aimed at reducing the burden of expensive health and personal care of older relatives for their families, and these innovative programs are meant to provide more options for Singaporeans in addition to the ones that already exist.

The fourth policy issue concerns the need to nurture leaders and managers with vision and creativity. Problem solving in creative and cost-effective ways will be a major challenge to voluntary welfare bodies because demand for managerial staff exceeds the supply in many areas. Further, the spirit of voluntarism in Singapore is relatively low compared to many western countries. With less than 10% of the population involved in voluntary activities, it will be necessary to recruit more volunteers for community-based programs. One step toward this goal was the setting up of a National Volunteer Centre in 1998 to coordinate and promote the spirit of voluntarism. The healthy young old, those aged 55-65 years, are a potential target group to involve, bearing in mind their ability to empathize with problems of old age.

The fifth area for policy attention is the need for more research and data on the future needs of elderly cohorts. Both quantitative and qualitative data are needed to assist the process of planning of appropriate services and programs for future decades. Thus far, the emphasis has been on health and financial needs. However, social care must be factored in if a comprehensive plan is to be put in place for the future. This task is more challenging because social needs are more difficult to project.

CONCLUSION

The future of long-term care in Singapore will be shaped by the extent to which the recommendations of the IMC are implemented.

The announcement made by the Minister for Community Development and Sports at the opening of the Regional Gerontological Conference in January 2001, in which he outlined the Five-Year Masterplan of Elder Care Services, reflects the endorsement of a number of recommendations of the IMCs on Health Care and Ageing Population. In particular, the initiatives regarding Multi-Service Centres, community support for caregivers, and revamping of the funding formula for VWOs were emphasized.

The suggestions put forward in the IMC Reports first must be systematically examined by the government through its various ministries and, if feasible, implemented over the next five years as far as possible. The Singapore government has taken a different route from other countries, where policy challenges of preparing for an aging population are assigned to specific administrative bodies established for that purpose. Since Singapore is such a small country, geographically as well as population-wise, this path seems to be appropriate for its use, phased in over a specified time frame. The administrative functions of the IMC on Ageing Population are executed by the Elderly Development Division, which is located in the Ministry of Community Development and Sports.

Singapore has the advantage of a stable economic and political climate, a powerful factor in ensuring continuity of strategies and programs not only for economic development but also for social and health services. Since the aging challenge affects almost every sector of Singaporean society, the government has decided on a holistic response involving several ministries, voluntary welfare organizations, the private sector, and even aging families. While Singapore is not a welfare state, the government takes a leading role in framing social policy. Thus, not only does the government promote the attitude that the public should look upon aging as a personal responsibility, shared with their immediate families; it also seeks to provide a social infrastructure in which these responsibilities can be realized. In so doing, the Asian cultural ethos of communal reciprocity as a public good is harnessed as a way of positive response to the societal challenge of an aging society.

REFERENCES

Atchley, R. (2000). *Social Forces and Aging: An Introduction to Gerontology.* 9th Edition. Wadsworth: Singapore.

Austin, C. (1986). Case management in long-term care. In C. Meyer's *Social Work and Aging* (2nd Ed.). National Association of Social Workers. Silver Spring: MD.

Challis, D., & Davies, B. (1986). *Case Management in Community Care: An Evaluated Experiment in the Home Care of the Elderly.* Gower Publishing: Aldershot, UK.

Cheung, P.L. (1993). Population ageing in Singapore. *Asia Pacific Journal of Social Work,* Volume *3*(2): 77-89.

Economic and Social Commission for Asia and the Pacific (1996). *Population Ageing in Asia and the Pacific.* ESCAP, Bangkok, with Japanese Organisation for International Cooperation in Family Planning, Inc., Tokyo. United Nations: New York.

Gordon, D., & Donald, S. (1993). *Community Social Work, Older People and Informal Care: A Romantic Illusion?* Avebury: Aldershot, UK.

Greene, V.L., Ondrich, J., & Laditka, S. (1998). Can home care services achieve cost savings in long-term care for older people? *Journal of Gerontology, 53B*(4): 228-328.

Knodel, J., & Debavalya, N. (1997). Living arrangements and support among the elderly in South-East Asia: An introduction. *Asia-Pacific Population Journal, 12*(4): 5-16.

Kua, E.H. (1987). Psychological distress for families caring for frail elderly. *Singapore Medical Journal, 3*: 42-44.

Mehta, K. (2000). Caring for the elderly in Singapore. In W. Liu & H. Kendig (Eds.). *Who Should Give Care to the Elderly? An East-West Social Value Divide.* Singapore University Press: Singapore.

Ministry of Community Development (1998). *Because We Care: Guidelines for Community-Based Services for Elderly.* Ministry of Community Development: Singapore.

Ministry of Community Development. (1999b). *Report of the Inter-Ministerial Committee on the Ageing Population.* Ministry of Community Development: Singapore.

Ministry of Health (1984). *Report of the Committee on the Problems of the Aged.* Ministry of Health: Singapore.

Ministry of Health (1999a). *Report of the Inter-Ministerial Committee on Health Care for the Elderly.* Ministry of Health: Singapore.

Ministry of Health, Ministry of Community Development, Department of Statistics and National Council of Social Services (1996). *National Survey of Senior Citizens in Singapore.* National Press: Singapore.

Pelham, A., & Clark, W. (Eds.) (1986). *Managing Home Care for the Elderly.* Springer Publishing: New York.

Prescott, N. (Ed.) (1998). *Proceedings of a Conference on Choices in Financing Health Care and Old Age Security.* World Bank Discussion Paper No. 2. World Bank. Washington, DC: USA.

Richards, M. (1996). *Community Care for Older People: Rights, Remedies and Finances.* Jordans: Bristol, UK.

Schneider, R., Kropf, N., & Kisor, A. (2000). *Gerontological Social Work: Knowledge, Service Settings, and Special Populations.* Brooks/Cole: Australia.

Shantakumar, G. (1994). *The Aged Population of Singapore.* Census of Population 1990, Monograph No. 1, Singapore.

Shantakumar, G. (1995). Aging and social policy in Singapore. *Ageing International,* 22(2): 49-54.

Siegel, J.S., & Hoover, S.L. (1982). Demographic aspects of health of the elderly to the year 2000 and beyond. *World Health Statistics Quarterly,* 35(3/4): 140-141.

Singapore Action Group of Elders (SAGE) (1998). *Case Management Service.* SAGE: Singapore.

Straits Times (1998). *Committee's 21 Members Named.* Singapore, November 15.

Teo, P. (1994). The national policy on elderly people in Singapore. *Ageing and Society,* 14: 405-427.

World Health Organization (1995). *World Health Report, 1995. Bridging the Gaps.* WHO: Geneva.

Exploring Policy and Financing Options for Long-Term Care in Taiwan

Shyh-Dye Lee, MD, MPH

Director/Chair, Graduate Institute of Long-Term Care
National Taipei College of Nursing

SUMMARY. Policy and financing arrangements for long-term care are important themes in each country and/or region, and Taiwan, with its unique historic and politico-economic background, can be regarded as a bridge between well-developed and under-developed countries. Policy formulation about long-term care in Taiwan involves several agencies in the government, including Ministry of Health, Interior Affairs, Education, Insurance Bureau, and Economic Council, and formulation of policy objectives has progressed considerably in the last five years. Financing arrangements are less well-developed because the National

Dr. Shyh-Dye Lee chairs the Advisory Council of Long-Term Care of the Ministry/Department of Health in Taiwan. He is also the Director/Chair of the Graduate Institute of Long-Term Care, National Taipei College of Nursing, and Chief/Director of the Division of Community Medicine at the Department of Family Medicine, National Taiwan University Hospital. He received his MD from National Taiwan University in 1982 and his Masters in Public Health from Johns Hopkins University in 1994. Dr. Lee is the recipient of the National Health Medal from the Ministry/Department of Health for Outstanding Work on Research at WONCA Asia Pacific Conference. He is also Chief Editor of the *Journal of Long Term Care* in Taiwan and an editorial board member for the *International Journal of Gerontology* in Japan.

Dr. Lee can be contacted at the Graduate Institute of Long-Term Care, National Taipei College of Nursing, 83-1 Nei-Chiang St., Taipei 108, Taiwan (E-mail: sdlee@ha.mc.ntu.edu.tw).

[Haworth co-indexing entry note]: "Exploring Policy and Financing Options for Long-Term Care in Taiwan." Lee, Shyh-Dye. Co-published simultaneously in *Journal of Aging & Social Policy* (The Haworth Press, Inc.) Vol. 13, No. 2/3, 2001, pp. 203-216; and: *Long-Term Care in the 21st Century: Perspectives from Around the Asia-Pacific Rim* (ed: Iris Chi, Kalyani K. Mehta, and Anna L. Howe) The Haworth Press, Inc., 2001, pp. 203-216. Single or multiple copies of this article are available for a fee from The Haworth Document Delivery Service [1-800-HAWORTH, 9:00 a.m. - 5:00 p.m. (EST). E-mail address: getinfo@haworthpressinc.com].

203

Health Insurance Program began only in 1995, and most long-term care is not yet covered. As demand for long-term care exceeds supply, and this gap will grow in future, current resource allocation measures are concerned to facilitate the expansion of community care rather than allowing institutional care to absorb more resources. Developing future financing options is now a central task for policymaking, and government must continue to take a leading role in consolidating financing and integrating the service systems. *[Article copies available for a fee from The Haworth Document Delivery Service: 1-800-HAWORTH. E-mail address: <getinfo@haworthpressinc.com> Website: <http://www.HaworthPress.com> © 2001 by The Haworth Press, Inc. All rights reserved.]*

KEYWORDS. Community care, financing arrangements, social insurance, Taiwan, veterans

THE POLICY CONTEXT

Taiwan is a modern industrial island country with a sophisticated historic and politico-economic status. Policymaking occurs mainly at the national government level, and in recent years, the concentration on economic policy has been balanced by increasing attention to social policy. The attention being given to aged care policy is part of this trend.

Since World War II, the economy of Taiwan has grown rapidly, and the standard of living has improved greatly. Per capita national income in 1996 was NT$321,174 (US$11,696), a ten-fold increase over the figure for 1976 (Directorate-General of Budget, 1997). Several indicators show that economic growth has been accompanied by social development. In 1976, only 7.4% of the adult population had any higher education, and the literacy rate was 85%; in 1995 it was estimated that 18% of the adult population had a higher education, and the literacy rate reached 94% (Ministry of Education, 1997). The proportion of the population enrolled in social security programs has increased from only some 4% when the programs began in 1956 to 13% by 1976, and by 1996, this figure had risen to 93%, or almost universal coverage.

The Ministry of Health was established in the Cabinet in March 1971, to manage health matters for the entire country, and the Bureau of National Health Insurance was set up on January 1, 1995 (Ministry of Health, 1998a; Ministry of Health & NHIB, 1994, 1995). Total health and medical care expenditure of governments at all levels in FY 1995 was NT$42.626 billion (approximately US$1.6 billion). Government and private sources are combined in "revolving funds" for medical care institutions at all levels, and in FY 1995 these totaled NT$52.694 billion (US$1.915 billion). The proportion of GNP spent on health care now stands at 4.7%. There are 115 doctors per 100,000 population and just four acute hospital beds per 1,000 population. Against these figures, until 1997, the provision of only 3.6 places in nursing homes and chronic care hospitals per 1,000 persons aged 65 years and over gives an indication of the very limited development of long-term care. However, the capacity of institutionalized care has been expanding with concerted policymaking in recent years, and, optimistically, will largely meet the need by 2005.

POLICY OBJECTIVES

Policy formulation in long-term care has progressed considerably in Taiwan in the last five years with the release of a number of policy reports from the Ministry of Interior Affairs (1997) and the Economic Progress Council (1996), together with a number of planning studies (Lee et al., 1995; Wu, Lue, & Lu, 1998; Wu et al., 1999) and research reports (Lee et al., 1995). Broad policy objectives can now be stated with reference to five areas.

The first objective is to address the rapid growth of those in need of care. As a higher proportion of the population reaches advanced ages, the number of older people who need assistance in personal care and activities of daily living will increase significantly. The burden of caring for the rapidly increasing number of elderly persons presents a formidable challenge to their families, to health care providers, to the government, and to the community at large.

The extent of current need is seen in a national survey of health and functional status conducted in 1996 (Ministry of Interior Affairs, 1997). Just over 5% of the older population, 100,000 people, reported a need for long-term care. The prevalence of ADL limitations in the community ranged from 2.4% to 5.4% for different activities; the most prevalent need reported is with bathing, and the least prevalent is for assistance with eating. The prevalence of ADL limitations is much higher in institutions, ranging from 28% to 81% for different activities (Ministry of Interior Affairs, 1997).

The second objective is to respond to the changing patterns of disease associated with a rapidly aging population. The ways in which the shift to chronic conditions, requiring a shift from cure to care-oriented services, and the sharp increase of the need for long-term care that has affected individuals, households, communities, and the whole society, have been well documented (WHO, 1997, 1999; Lee et al., 1995; Lee, 1996; Wu, Lue, & Lu, 1998; Wu et al., 1999). At a practical level, health and social care services must adapt to help the elderly or patients with bio-psycho-social handicaps and assist them in achieving self-care and autonomy, enhancing their esteem and dignity, and thereby lessening the load on society and countering concerns of social security and welfare.

As well as responding to changing patterns of use of health care, services will have to take account of living arrangements in responding to the increasing need for personal care and coping with functional limitations. The third objective, therefore, is to recognize that models of family care must be developed to maintain the traditional patterns that still hold in living arrangements for the elderly in Taiwan. Almost three out of four older people live with their children, and almost one in five lives with his or her spouse; less than 3% live in long-term care facilities and 1.4% in apartments for the elderly (Ministry of Interior Affairs, 1997).

As care for the elderly is still supervised and regulated separately by two government systems and two sets of agencies, the fourth policy objective is to overcome this division. The Ministry of Health takes charge of health care issues for the elderly, while the Ministry of Interior Affairs deals with personal care and daily living services. This division of responsibility constitutes a major barrier in policymaking and results in difficulties in organizing and administering aged care services.

The fifth objective is to systemize financing of long-term care. At present, there is some sporadic public funding that supports some particular parts of the social welfare and the veterans' systems. However, most long-term care services are bought and paid for out-of-pocket by individuals or families when care or service is necessary and actually used. While financing arrangements for long-term care, such as social insurance, can only proceed after the pension system has been set up and related facilities have been prepared, policy development is needed now to ensure that financing arrangements are consistent with the development and funding of the service delivery system.

It is now accepted that the long-term care delivery system must be mandated and established as soon as possible. In addition, developments in related fields, such as education and training, development of geriatric medicine and gerontology, and health care research, are recognized as necessary to address the urgent need for assistance in policy decision-making, administration, monitoring, and evaluation. These policy development processes are similar to those experienced in many other countries and regions (WHO, 1997, 1999; Lee et al., 1995; OECD, 1996).

ROLES OF GOVERNMENT

A number of structures are in place for long-term care policymaking. Within the Ministry of Health, there is an Advisory Committee on Long-Term

Care, the National Health Insurance Bureau (NHIB) administers the national health insurance program, and the National Health Research Institutes include a Division of Geriatrics and Gerontology (Ministry of Health, 2000; Ministry of Health & NHIB, 1996; Lee et al., 1995). Geriatric medicine is included in the program of the Department of Medicine and Community Health at several general hospitals, such as the National Taiwan University Hospital and some other medical centers; and the National Taipei College of Nursing has set up the first Graduate Institute of Long-Term Care in Taiwan. Contributions to policy discussion are also made by the Gerontological Society and Long-Term Care Professional Association of Taiwan, which publish the *Journal of Long-Term Care* in Taiwan. The author is involved in these different bodies in a variety of roles (Lee, 2000).

The Council for Elderly Welfare comes under the Ministry of Interior Affairs, which is responsible for welfare policy and so concerned with subsidizing special facilities and special subgroups, such as those in poverty, and the low- to mid-income population. The veterans' system provides pensions, subsidies, and allowances for healthy veterans to meet their daily living needs as well as providing long-term care facilities.

These divisions in government responsibility run parallel to the division of the service delivery system into four segments: the medical care system, social welfare system, retired servicemen's or veterans' system, and private sectors. Policymaking is proceeding on two main fronts to overcome this divided system. First, integration of the medical care, social welfare, and veterans' systems is seen as inevitable, and planning for the development of a comprehensive and continuing long-term care program has commenced. A Coordinating Council for Elderly Care has been established to hold periodic meetings and provide for operating linkages between the Ministry of Health, Ministry of Interior Affairs, and the Vocational Assistance Commission for Retired Servicemen. Second, a number of amendments have been made to acts and laws relating to long-term care, including the Elderly Welfare Act, the Medical Practice Act, and Nurses' Law. Regulations, standards, and criteria for procedures and conditions for operating institutional services have been relaxed with a view to facilitating the setting up of services and fostering the expansion of the long-term care delivery system.

CURRENT FINANCING ARRANGEMENTS

The National Health Insurance Program (NHIP) was started in March 1995, under the National Health Insurance Act. A preventive health care service for the elderly under this program was started in April 1996 (Ministry of Health &

NHIB, 1994, 1995). To ease the financial burden, the population covered by the NHIP was then required to meet a limited part of health and care expenditures.

NHIP is funded by premiums paid at large. Citizens, employers, and government contribute shares of 40%, 50%, and 10%, respectively, to the premiums. Families of those in the workforce are covered with the upper limit of five persons per family in the past, but shifting to three currently. However, the self-employed must carry the major share of the premiums, contributing 90%. Payment of premiums is compulsory for all people, including the elderly, and the only exemptions are the low-income group and centenarians in the capital area. The premium has been set at an upper limit of 4.25% of income. The sharing of 90% of the premiums between the population and employers means that government must provide 10% from general revenue. The National Health Insurance Bureau is the single agency in charge of administering the NHIP, and other groups, such as employer or employee organizations, can play only secondary roles (Ministry of Health & NHIB, 1994, 1995).

Most long-term care is not as yet funded by the NHIP. Only a very limited part of services provided in chronic care hospitals and professional medical nursing care in a long-term care package (nursing home care and home-based nursing care) is now covered. Long-term care was ignored by policymakers at the beginning of the NHIP, and while an investigation into the feasibility of covering long-term care was made subsequently by the Ministry of Health and National Health Insurance Bureau (1996), the very substantial resource commitments precluded any action being taken.

Review of payments made by the NHIP for long-term care has lead to three developments. First, following a pilot project of payment for home care by the Government Employee's Insurance, home care payments were included in the National Health Insurance Program. Second, research is underway into the feasibility of payment schedules for different services, and related preparatory work is proceeding, such as studying the cost-effectiveness of home care of respiratory-dependent patients, discharge planning for chronic patients, and the establishment of service models for hospice care. Third, the results of these studies are being taken up in the formulation of long-term care policy; the NHIP coverage of professional medical nursing care as part of a long-term care package came about in this way.

Older people and their families must meet most of the cost of long-term care privately or through related means, for example, self-payment (self-insurance), support or supplementation from siblings or other relatives. There is also some sporadic use of home equity conversion (reverse mortgage or similar), commercial insurance, small tax credits, and some non-official provident funds, but these options are very limited. So far, there is still no reliable database on the proportions of expenditure each covers as the social welfare system remunerates some kinds of consumption of long-term care for the low-income group only.

RESOURCE ALLOCATION

The central or core problem of long-term care policy and delivery in Taiwan is one of resource allocation: demand cannot be effectively met by the existing supply of services. There is a lack of manpower, whether professional, semi-professional, or non-professional, and of facilities, so families, especially women, must take responsibility for care for the elderly and the disabled. A further problem is the imbalance in provision and use of hospital and other institutional care. Elderly patients or patients with chronic conditions occupy acute or sub-acute beds, so that all facilities are fully occupied in the medical care system and the social welfare system. Unregistered facilities such as homes for the elderly and other care institutions appeared and grew rapidly until 1999 when regulations started to take effect. At the same time, due to natural attrition and other trends, there is a vacancy rate of around 20% in the veterans' system, especially in the eastern and southern parts of Taiwan (Ministry of Interior Affairs, 1997; Ministry of Health, 1997).

To provide appropriate and accessible long-term care services, a number of tasks must be undertaken to establish the policy framework for the long-term care delivery system. First of all, it is necessary to define and present the problems that are to be dealt with. Second, the scale of these problems and the magnitude of their impacts must be measured; as well as analyzing the determinants of these problems, projections of future trends must be made. The final task is to set priorities and evaluate options. Progress has been made with these tasks in the development of a number of direct resource allocation measures and indirect measures that offer incentives for providers to develop long-term care services (Lee et al., 1995; Lee, 1996, 1998).

Today, the NHIP scheme partially covers long-term care service delivery, and it may extend as far as is possible within the medical care part of long-term care (Ministry of Health, 2000; Ministry of Health & NHIB, 1996).

The focus on home-based and community-based care, which currently accounts for some 75% of long-term care capacity, must be maintained rather than allowing institution-based care to increase above its present 25% share. However, there is still no actual systematized funding base for institutional or community care. To this end, more funds are needed to improve the welfare of the elderly by subsidizing their living expenses and subsidizing the costs of their nursing and medical care in addition to payments made by the National

Health Insurance Program. Service hours and fee scales for home care also must be adjusted upwards to provide for the elderly of middle and low-income families. Additional financing arrangements, such as medical savings accounts and auxiliary social insurance, are under consideration (Ministry of Interior Affairs, 1997; Lee, 1998; Ministry of Health, 2000; Ministry of Health & NHIB, 1996; Tseng, 1998).

Facilitating outreach services from the public-sector institutions, in competition in the market for acute and sub-acute care, can also contribute to maintaining the lead of community-based care, as can augmenting the limited number of health stations and community service or welfare centers that currently exist. Referral and follow-up systems for long-term care that can be promoted as working models for discharge planning for chronic patients, are also being initiated and adopted in acute care. Expansion of subsidized access to assistive devices will also facilitate community-based care, together with subsidies for the maintenance, modification, and reconstruction of residences to make them more suitable for the elderly with functional handicaps. Finally, 11 demonstration centers for long-term care, on a single point of entry model, will be set up and supported for an outreach approach providing assessment of long-term care needs, managing health care, arranging assistive devices and counseling, and providing operational support (Ministry of Health, 1997, 2000).

Another set of measures is directed to achieving a better balance of resources used for long-term care, and the establishment of both home care and care institutions is being encouraged. In the first instance, support can be given to organizations providing long-term care by clearly defining the types of functions they are to provide as nursing homes, personal care, home care, nursing care, and day care. As well as subsidizing home care, subsidies made available to public and private homes for the elderly that provide only basic care can convert the homes to care institutions. Attention is also being given to networking long-term care service delivery and the service information system, to link separate services together and provide information on services (Ministry of Health, 1997, 2000).

Three measures aim to provide incentives for providers to expand long-term care services by reducing their costs. First, separate and less stringent regulation of care workers in long-term institutions means that staffing is less costly than in acute hospitals. Second, tax reductions are being considered for nursing care institutions (nursing homes and similar ones) and amendments to land use regulation could also ease costs. Third, arrangements for collecting care fees, and controls over the use of these payments, are being relaxed to give greater freedom to nursing homes affiliated with hospitals, especially in the public sectors, so that hospital superintendents or core personnel are able to employ additional nursing and other care staff in their affiliated nursing facilities (Ministry of Health, 2000; Tseng, 1998).

Several measures are being taken to reorient some acute hospital services towards long-term care. The Medical Development Fund will subsidize the interest on loans for up to 15 years to encourage registered, private-sector organizations to set up facilities for long-term care of the chronically ill. The focus is on nursing care institutions rather than medical care institutions, which were the main focus in the past. Further, a plan is in place to evaluate the use of vacant beds in the veterans system to make the best use of these resources (Ministry of Health, 1997, 2000; Lee, 1996).

Initiatives are also being taken to develop models of care for the dying and for those with severe handicaps. These include starting to plan for hospice care and conducting a pilot project in hospice care institutions using payments by the NHIP. Hospitals are also being encouraged to develop shared care models, home care, outreach community care, institutional care, and special care for respirator-dependent patients and patients with other severe chronic conditions (Ministry of Health, 1997, 2000; Lee, 1996).

The long-term care workforce is being enhanced by incorporating relevant courses into the curricula of nursing education and practice as required subjects, and training courses are being organized for medical and welfare workers, and for care providers in teaching hospitals and nursing homes. Regulations and systems concerning the licensing of long-term care personnel are also being set up to enhance training of managers or administrators of nursing care institutions. Action is also being taken to secure the cooperation of professional associations in facilitating continuing medical education and training for physicians, nurses, social workers, and health care practitioners in other disciplines, such as occupational therapists, physical therapists, nutritionists, and other professionals in geriatrics, hospice care, and general care of the elderly and chronically ill patients (Lee, 1996; Ministry of Health, 1997, 2000).

Finally, systems for quality control and assurance are being organized through evaluation, monitoring, and supervision to improve the quality of long-term care services. These measures include development of operating procedures and guidelines for service models, setting up demonstration centers, and publishing a manual on the design and construction of nursing homes. International communication is prompted by inviting international experts to join seminars and symposiums to advance experience, knowledge, and skills. Finally, an accreditation and monitoring system for quality control and quality assurance is being initiated. Monitoring of unlicensed care institutions is also being strengthened, especially since the validation of the Elderly Welfare Act after June 18, 1999 (Lee, 1996; Ministry of Health, 1997).

FUTURE FINANCING OPTIONS

As Prescott (1999) has argued, decisions about financing arrangements are more critical in setting up and operating the long-term care system than demographic trends or health care needs. The comprehensiveness of financing arrangements is the predominant determinant of the feasibility and likely success of the future delivery of long-term care. Organizing the financing arrangements is the basic policy task, and it is essential for the development of the service delivery system to be accompanied by detailed, accurate, and prospective financial calculations (Prescott, 1999; Gujarati, 1995; Tseng, 1998).

In planning incoming financial arrangements, consideration must be given to a possible combination or package of the following (Ministry of Health, 1997; Tseng, 1998):

- Social insurance, along the lines of U. S. Medicare or Singapore's Medishield;
- A budget allocation from taxes to subsidize institutional care services, local social services, and cash benefits;
- Public pensions;
- Private medical care saving accounts, business insurance; and
- Self-payment of out-of-pocket expenses.

In line with the general view expressed by Prescott (1999), Tseng has seen social insurance as playing the predominant role in reducing the potential risk of financial burden, and the remainder as supplementary or auxiliary options for Taiwan, where the highest priority in financing arrangements for the long-term care system has been stated as assuring its "maintenance forever" (Tseng, 1998).

According to the experiences reported for OECD countries, the percentage of GDP spent on long-term care can be regarded as a significant indicator in policymaking (OECD, 1996). The first practical step is to estimate the financial burden in relation to GDP. At present, the cost of the broad spectrum of long-term care for the elderly in Taiwan is approximately 0.27% of GDP, or US$0.83 billion. The share for institution-based care is around 0.11% of GDP, or US$0.34 billion, about 40% of the total government expenditure on long-term care. However, closer scrutiny of the content of long-term care suggests that institution-based care accounts for only 29% of all expenditure at present, and 71% is accounted for by home-based care, of which 62% is by families, relatives, or friends; 3% comes from the social welfare system, and 6% from the medical care system. Community-based services at present account for less than 0.5% of total expenditure (Directorate-General of Budget, 1997; Economic Progress Council, 1996; Tseng, 1998).

Estimates also must be made of the potential costs of expansion of the long-term care system, which is currently growing at around 5% per year, and related to projected growth of GDP to determine the share to pour into long-term care issues. The experience from the OECD member countries in the proportion of GDP spent on long-term care may provide a reference for Taiwan (Sundstrom, 1994; Gujarati, 1995; Tseng, 1998). Consideration of current and projected demographic structure needs to take account not only of the percentage of elderly in the population and possible improvements in life expectancy, but also the percentage of the elderly who are disabled or unable to care for themselves (Sundstrom, 1994; Tseng, 1998).

Changes in utilization of different care systems also must be estimated. It is considered that home-based family care will fall from 65% to 45% over the next 20 years, with community-based care increasing from 5% to 25%. Institution-based care will be held at around 30% (Ministry of Health, 1998a, 1998b; Ministry of Interior Affairs, 1997).

The combination or package of different financing arrangements most suited to Taiwan's needs is currently being studied. The number, criteria, and methods of payments for home care services are being reviewed, together with planning for inclusion of long-term care in the National Health Insurance Program (Ministry of Health & NHIB, 1996; Ministry of Health; 1997).

In studying additional long-term care insurance, the level of the premium and the ways of sharing contributions must be planned. Payment schedules for various care needs and methods of payment have to be investigated, including cash payments, cash allowances, or service payments, and whether or not the needs of informal caregivers should also be attended to. Recommendations on the feasibility, timing, and methods of developing long-term care insurance also must address coordination between long-term care insurance and the pension system (Ministry of Health, 1997).

Past experience and current conditions in the OECD countries demonstrate the common adoption of financial arrangements combining at least two systems, with differences among countries in the proportions that each makes up (Sundstrom, 1994; OECD, 1996). Just as in the European cases, the Taiwanese pension system could in future be joined with long-term care insurance, or long-term care insurance could accompany medical savings accounts. Tax funding could be used to aid the poor, low-income, deprived, or under-served groups. If a social insurance program is adopted as the financing arrangement for long-term care, four possibilities are available: an independent social insurance program, incorporation into the NHIP as a compulsory additional insurance program, or as a voluntary additional insurance program, or incorporation into the general medical insurance system (Tseng, 1998).

As the pension system is just now being planned and organized, Wu, Tseng, and others working on the development of social insurance for long-term care regard it as a long and winding path to follow, but one that may ultimately lead to a satisfactory outcome for financing and service delivery by supporting the supply of manpower and development of facilities (Wu, Lue, & Lu, 1998; Tseng, 1998; Wu et al., 1999).

THE WAY AHEAD

In looking into the future, it is apparent that government must continue to play an active role in designing, developing, and establishing the framework for policymaking and financing of long-term care in Taiwan. It must exercise its mandate to estimate the need for long-term care accurately and integrate the different systems that currently provide long-term care systems for the elderly. Government must manage the shifts in demand generated by demographic trends, the level of expenditure and proportion of GDP to be allocated to long-term care, and the distribution of long-term care facilities and their utilization by the elderly. As well as creating resources for long-term care, government must assist directly and indirectly in many areas, including setting up facilities, nurturing manpower, and weaving the strands of the delivery system together. In consolidating the financing basis for long-term care, consideration is being given to adding social insurance to existing arrangements.

While the initiatives just presented had been progressing quietly for some time, policy development was significantly advanced in the formal approval of the integrated Three-Year Plan for the Long-Term Care of the Elderly on July 1, 1998, to run until June 30, 2001, when it was reevaluated. A three-year pilot project for establishing the long-term care delivery system for the elderly was subsequently launched, to run until December 31, 2004 (Ministry of Health, 1997). As part of the Plan, it is intended to carry out the pilot project as an empirical trial. One community will be selected in each of an urban, rural, and aboriginal area to establish a long-term care system and put it into practical operation. These pilot projects will incorporate institutional care, community-based care, home health care including home care and home nursing, dementia care, respite care, and so on. The outcomes of the pilot projects and the Plan overall will be reviewed in three years time and will have a major influence on the future direction of long-term care in Taiwan.

REFERENCES

Directorate-General of Budget (1997). *Accounting and Statistics (Taiwan): National Income of Taiwan*. Taipei: Directorate-General of Budget, Accounting and Statistics, Executive Yuan.

Economic Progress Council, Taiwan (1996). *Population Estimates 1995-2036*. Taipei: Economic Progression Council, Executive Yuan.

Gujarati, D. N. (1995). *Basic Econometrics*, 3rd edition. New York: McGraw-Hill, International Edition.

Lee, S. D. (2000). *Long-Term Care Issues in Taiwan (Update)*. Taipei: Annual Congress of Gerontological Society of Taiwan.

Lee, S. D. (1998). Health and care for the elderly. *Journal of Long-Term Care, 2*(1): 1-6.

Lee, S. D. (1996). Health care and policy for the elderly. *J Reh Med, 4*(1): S1-4.

Lee, S. D., Kuo, J. S. et al. (1995). *Planning Report of Gerontological Research, National Health Research Institutes*. Taipei: Planning Group of Gerontological Research, Division of Gerontological Research, National Health Research Institutes (NHRI).

Ministry of Education, Taiwan (1997). *Statistical Indices of Education*. Taipei: Ministry of Education, Executive Yuan.

Ministry of Health, Taiwan (2000). *Annual Report of Public Health in Taiwan–1999*. Taipei: Ministry of Health, Executive Yuan.

Ministry of Health, Taiwan (1998a). *Annual Report of Public Health in Taiwan–1997*. Taipei: Ministry of Health, Executive Yuan.

Ministry of Health, Taiwan (1998b). *General Health Statistics in Taiwan*. Taipei: Ministry of Health, Executive Yuan.

Ministry of Health, Taiwan (1997). *Three-Year Plan for the Long-Term Care of the Elderly*. Taipei: Ministry of Health, Executive Yuan.

Ministry of Health & National Health Insurance Bureau, Taiwan (1996). *Evaluation Report on the Feasibility of Long-Term Care Consumption Covered by National Health Insurance Program*. Taipei: Ministry of Health & National Health Insurance Bureau (Taiwan).

Ministry of Health & National Health Insurance Bureau, Taiwan (1994-95). *National Health Insurance Act (with related Regulations, Rules, Standards, Criterion)*. Taipei: Ministry of Health & National Health Insurance Bureau.

Ministry of Interior Affairs, Taiwan (1997*). Surveillance Report of Elderly Related Issues–1996*. Taipei: Ministry of Interior Affairs, Executive Yuan.

OECD (1996). *Caring for Frail Elderly People: Policies in Evolution*. Paris: OECD.

Prescott, N. (Ed.) (1996). Proceedings of a Conference on Choices in Financing Health Care and Old Age Security. *World Bank Discussion Paper*. No. 2. Washington, DC: World Bank.

Sundstrom, G. (1994). Care by the families: An overview of trends, in OECD (1994), *Caring for Frail Elderly People: New Direction in Care*. Paris: OECD.

Tseng, C. N. (1998). *The Structuring of 5th Social Insurance Blueprint–A Study on the Allocation of Insurance Resources for the Long-Term Care*. Masters Degree Thesis, Graduate Institute of Social Welfare, Chung-Cheng University.

World Health Organization (WHO) (1997). *World Health Statistics Annual.* Geneva: WHO.

World Health Organization (WHO) (1999). *Ageing and Health: A Global Challenge for the 21st Century.* Kobe, Japan: WHO Center for Health Development.

Wu, S. C., Lue, P. C., & Lu, R. F. (1998). *The Study on the Long-Term Care Policy–Following Social Welfare System in Taiwan.* Taipei: Research & Accredit Council, Executive Yuan.

Wu, S. C., Wang, C., Lin, W. Y., Wu, Y. C., & Wang, R. C. (1999). *Ten-Year Plan for the Establishment of Long-Term Care System for the Elderly in Taiwan.* Taipei: Executive Yuan.

Organization and Delivery
of Long-Term Care in Taiwan

Herng-Chia Chiu, PhD

Kaohsiung Medical University, Taiwan

SUMMARY. Taiwan reached the World Health Organization (WHO) benchmark of 7% aged 65 and over for defining an aging population only as recently as 1993. With this proportion projected to double to 14% by 2020, Taiwan faces a rapid increase in need for long-term care. This article presents an account of the current service delivery system, which is divided between health and social affairs administrations, with a substantial role also taken by the Veteran Administration, and growing provision of facilities that operate outside the government-registered system. While a basic level of both institutional and community care services has developed, they are not organized into an integrated service system. Problems arising from the divisions and overlaps in responsibility are identified in relation to competition for resources, differences in regulation and eligibility, funding arrangements and misallocation of resources, and divergent views about the philosophical basis of long-term care. Other aspects of services fall under each jurisdiction, but there is

---

Dr. Herng-Chia Chiu is Director of the Department of Medical Records in Kaohsiung Medical University. He received his PhD in health service research at Virginia Commonwealth University. He has been Chairperson, Committee of Long-Term Care Planning, Kaohsiung City, and Board Member of the Chinese Long-Term Care Professional Association since 1997 and 1996, respectively. He has published a number of papers in journals about long-term care in Taiwan.

Dr. Chiu can be contacted at 100 Shih-Chun 1st Rd., Department of Public Health, Kaohsiung, Taiwan, 807 (E-mail: chiu@cc.kmc.edu.tw).

[Haworth co-indexing entry note]: "Organization and Delivery of Long-Term Care in Taiwan." Chiu, Herng-Chia. Co-published simultaneously in *Journal of Aging & Social Policy* (The Haworth Press, Inc.) Vol. 13, No. 2/3, 2001, pp. 217-232; and: *Long-Term Care in the 21st Century: Perspectives from Around the Asia-Pacific Rim* (ed: Iris Chi, Kalyani K. Mehta, and Anna L. Howe) The Haworth Press, Inc., 2001, pp. 217-232. Single or multiple copies of this article are available for a fee from The Haworth Document Delivery Service [1-800-HAWORTH, 9:00 a.m. - 5:00 p.m. (EST). E-mail address: getinfo@haworthpressinc.com].

217

also some overlap. A case study of Taiwan's second largest city, Kaohsiung City, reports the outcomes of these divisions as a thin spread of a range of services rather than a coordinated service network. Several planning exercises have been undertaken in recent years to address these problems, and although at an early stage of implementation, the outcomes of these plans are seen as shaping the future directions of long-term care in Taiwan. *[Article copies available for a fee from The Haworth Document Delivery Service: 1-800-HAWORTH. E-mail address: <getinfo@haworthpressinc.com> Website: <http://www.HaworthPress.com> © 2001 by The Haworth Press, Inc. All rights reserved.]*

KEYWORDS. Taiwan, veterans, service fragmentation, family caregivers, adult day care, respite care, eligibility

TAIWAN'S AGING POPULATION

Aging is a universal phenomenon of increasing importance to both developed and developing countries as their older populations increase. Comparison with other nations in Asia shows that Taiwan is not alone in the rapid increase of the elderly population. In Taiwan, only 2.4% of the population was aged 65 and over in the 1950s, but this proportion had doubled by the 1980s, and in 1993 surpassed the 7% mark set by the World Health Organization (WHO) as denoting an "aged population."

As of 1999, the elderly population of 1.82 million accounted for 8.3% of the total population of 21.74 million. Life expectancy has increased markedly over the last 50 years and now stands at 71.9 years for men and 77.8 years for women; at age 65, further life expectancy is 16.6 years for men and 19.3 years for women. The even gender balance of Taiwan's older population, with a slight excess of males, 51%, is atypical for an aging population and is due to historical events that saw large numbers of soldiers and refugees withdraw to Taiwan in 1949.

It is projected that the elderly population of Taiwan will reach 14% by year 2020 (Council for Economic Planning and Development, 2000). The proportion of aged will have doubled in just 21 years, and the absolute number of older people will have increased by 90%. With a higher proportion of the population reaching advanced ages, the number of older people who need assistance in personal care and daily activities will increase significantly. As a consequence, the burden of caring for the rapidly increasing number of elderly presents a formidable challenge to their families, to health care providers, to the government, and to the community at large.

The growth of the elderly population in Taiwan has evolved along with changes in society. The success of industrialization has changed not only economic structures but social structures as well. As in many other Asian countries, mainly families, friends, and neighbors care for the elderly in Taiwan. According to the 1996 survey on living arrangements conducted by the Department of Internal Affairs, 73% of the elderly considered living with children as the ideal living arrangement, and 16% preferred to live with their spouses only. Just under 3% prefer to live in a residential long-term care facility, and 1.4% chose elderly apartments (Department of Statistics, Ministry of the Interior, 1996). These preferred living arrangements correspond closely to actual arrangements, and living at home with children is still the preferred and actual living arrangement for most of the elderly in Taiwan. How to take this preference into consideration for program development is a central task for Taiwan.

The Need for Long-Term Care

Any program for the elderly in Taiwan must be oriented to the realities of Taiwan, of daily life for Taiwanese senior citizens, and of their physical and psychosocial needs. While it is recognized that the need for long-term care stems from a variety of limitations in physical or mental abilities or in family and social support systems, very few studies in Taiwan have explored how many of the elderly population need long-term care from a multidimensional perspective.

The most popular and extensively used measurement scale is the index of Activities of Daily Living (ADL), which includes basic ADL items covering eating, bathing, dressing, using toilet, and physical movement, and instrumental IADL items. On the basis of surveys measuring ADLs, it had been estimated that approximately 106,201 persons were in need of long-term care at the end of 1997 (Department of Health, 1998). Among them, 95,590 persons were aged 65 or over, giving a prevalence of ADL limitation in 5.5% of the total elderly population in Taiwan. In addition to functional disability, chronic disease is another determinant of long-term care utilization. The major diagnoses for those currently receiving either home care or institutional care are cerebrovascular disease, diabetes, and dementia (Department of Health, 1998).

WHAT SERVICES ARE NEEDED AND PROVIDED?

One of the most difficult challenges in long-term care is translating a set of functional disabilities and assistance needs into a prescription for a package of services. Service delivery in Taiwan today reflects the efforts of governmental agencies, charitable organizations, and other individual agencies to address the challenge. The governmental agencies can be classified into three systems: the health care agencies under the Department of Health, social welfare agencies under the Department of Social Affairs, and the Veteran Administration. Each system had its own mechanisms and policies, creating different segments of long-term care that are poorly integrated and so fail to offer a continuum of care.

In terms of care settings, long-term care can be delivered in institutions, at home, and in the community (Brody & Masciocchi, 1980). Four types of institutions traditionally provide institutional care for the elderly in Taiwan: public homes for the aged, private homes for the aged, veteran hospital-based chronic units, and veteran homes. Social welfare agencies and the Veteran Administration fund all of these long-term care facilities, except for some of the private-sector homes for the aged. Long-term care facilities funded by the social welfare system admit only those elderly able to perform activities of daily living; this is in marked contrast to institutional care in other countries, and facilities providing independent living elsewhere are often part of the housing system rather than the long-term care system.

Long-term care programs under the health care system are provided through hospitals, chronic hospitals, nursing homes, and day care centers. The provision of health-related long-term services is guided by and administered under the Medical Practice Act, the Nurses' Act, and other relevant regulations. One segment of institutional care is not under any regulation, control, or management: the non-registered long-term care nursing homes. Most of these non-registered facilities are profit-oriented and claim to provide "skilled" nursing care but do not have sufficient nursing professionals. Quality of care thus needs close attention.

Home care refers to a wide variety of services for older and disabled persons who may not need nursing facility care but require some assistance with their day-to-day health and personal needs while living at home. Home care services fall into two categories: skilled care and home support services. Skilled nursing care is generally given under the direction of a physician and consists of health care by nurse practitioners, including but not limited to, home dialysis, nutrition services, and skilled nursing. In Taiwan, registered nurses employed by hospitals, home care agencies, and local health agencies provide most of the skilled nursing care. Home support services are highly personalized and include personal care and homemaker services. In most cases in Taiwan, the family provides home support, but more and more home services programs have been developed by social welfare agencies in recent years to assist families.

Community-based long-term care is provided in settings both inside and outside the home, usually in a more structured environment than the home support service component of home care. Examples of popular community-based services are Adult Day Health Care Centers, operated by hospitals or senior centers, and Senior Centers that provide activities such as long-life classes, sponsored by the social welfare departments and transportation services. Community-based care offers opportunities for older persons with disabilities to get together socially and participate in recreational activities, and also includes respite care for families and caregivers. While the basic array of home and community services is now established in Taiwan, other community-based long-term services, such as counseling, legal services, information and referral services, and congregate meal sites are still at early stages of development.

SERVICES AND PROGRAMS
PROVIDED BY THE SOCIAL WELFARE SYSTEM

Most types of long-term services or programs are provided under the authority of the social welfare system and the health care system, but there are some differences in eligibility and other aspects of delivery.

Home and Community Services

Home services and community-based long-term care services are very important in the continuum of care, and are primarily provided by the social welfare system in Taiwan. A distinction is made between home care and home services.

Home Care for the Chronically Disabled Aged. The major purpose of this program is to maintain the disabled elderly living in the community as long as possible with in-home assistance. Usually, a homemaker with minimum training in taking care of disabled persons will be sent to the home of disabled elderly who either have chronic physical or mental conditions, or have difficulty in carrying out activities of daily living. Families with an elder aged 65 and over who has a chronic condition are entitled to utilize the home care program. In addition, the total household income of eligible families must be at the lowest income level.

The service package delivered by the home care program includes assistance with eating, psychological consultation, hygiene, rehabilitation, and nutritional services. Most of the operating facilities for home help services are not-for-profit organizations, such as Taiwan Red Cross and the Taiwan Long-Life Association.

Home Services for the Aged. The home services program for the aged has a similar purpose to the home care program, but there is a major difference in eligibility. The home care program is not only limited to the elderly; recipients must also have a diagnosed chronic condition. On the other hand, the elderly who simply have difficulty in living at home are eligible for home services. Again, only legally approved persons or associations are eligible to provide home services programs, which include house cleaning, laundry, and health care assistance. It is expected that 400 community centers will qualify to provide home services programs (Department of Health, 1998).

Community-Based Services

Community-based long-term care services consist of adult day care, nutritional services, recreational services, life-long educational programs, respite care, and related services. Since adult day care and respite care programs are the most important, they are addressed further here.

Adult Day Care is a formally structured program of substitute care provided at hospital sites or in the community. Adult day care centers are most used by those older people who have families at home who need to work full-time. The families need a safe and friendly place to take care of their parents or relatives during the day and to provide social interaction. Taiwan's day care program is provided and funded by both social welfare and health care systems. The operating organizations can be hospitals or any interested groups with professional staff.

Respite Care or Short-Stay Program. The respite care program is an effort to provide temporary relief for the primary caregivers of the bedridden elderly by placing the older person in a nursing home for a short period. The fundamental goal of this program is to improve the quality of life for family members by reducing caregiver burden. Related respite care programs are also operated by the Department of Health long-term demonstration project and jointly funded by social welfare and health care agencies. The target set for the year 2000 is to provide respite for 1,000 persons (Department of Health, 1998).

In addition to formal services provided by different social welfare agencies, there are support groups for caregivers, mainly provided by a range of volunteer groups involved in community care in Taiwan. The Taiwan Association of Caregivers and Taiwan Long-Term Care Association are two examples of the efforts of volunteer organizations.

Institutional Care

There are three types of institutional settings under the supervision of the social welfare system, and non-registered long-term care facilities provide a similar range of services. Figures in Table 1 show the number of places in 1999 and 2000.

Homes for the Aged primarily accommodate healthy elderly who could not live at home because of economic status or social impairments. Persons aged 60 and above who live alone and whose household income level is below the poverty line are eligible to live in either public or private homes as long as there is space available. If the recipient uses a private-sector home, the local government will reimburse the expenses later. Homes for the aged are residential in nature, with the services provided by the home focusing on social and recreation activities. Some homes also have equipped themselves with health

TABLE 1. Types and Number of Long-Term Care Beds in Social Welfare and Health Care Systems

Types of long-term care facility	1999			2000		
	No.	No. of places		No.	No. of places	
Social welfare system (a)						
Home for aged (Public)	17	6,711		16	6,385	
Home for aged (Private)	38	5,249	11,960	37	5,738	12,123
Social nursing facility (Public)	16	1,573		17	1,695	
Social nursing facility (Private)	39	2,664	4,237	382	9,479	11,074
Non-registered nursing care facility (b)	446	20,865		n.a.	n.a.	
Health care system (c)						
Chronic hospital	15	4,691		15	4,691	
Freestanding NH	31	1,320		31	1,920	
Public hospital based NH	24	1,164	5,655	24	1,590	10,385
Private hospital based NH	77	3,171		77	6,875	
Veteran administration (d)						
Veteran home	14	15,870		14	15,279	
Veteran hospital based NH	11	390		11	1,310	

Source:
(a) Department of Social Affairs, Ministry of the Interior, Republic of China, 2000.
(b) Chiu et al., *Impacts of National Health Insurance on the Long-Term Care System*, Technical Report. Department of Health, Taipei.
(c) Department of Health, The Executive Yuan, Republic of China, Three-Year Plan for Long-Term Care of the Elderly, 1998.
(d) Statistics Department, Veterans Affairs Commission, The Executive Yuan, Republic of China, 2000.

or medical facilities. Home residents pay different levels of fees based on their financial status. In mid 2000, there were 53 homes for the aged listed with the social welfare system, and they accounted for 12,123 residential places.

Social Nursing Facilities provide similar care to nursing homes. The difference is that social nursing facilities come under the social welfare system rather than the health care system. Social nursing facilities admit older persons who need constant care due to pronounced physical or mental disabilities; the major diagnoses of the residents are dementia, stroke, and/or coma conditions. Low-income status is also a condition for eligibility for admission. After admission, residents are assessed periodically to evaluate their continuing eligibility.

Social nursing facilities must be registered and legally approved. The private sector dominates provision; at the end of 1999, there were 16 public social nursing facilities with 1,573 beds, and 39 private institutions with 2,664 beds. The total number of nursing home beds was expected to reach 11,074 at the end of 2000. In year 1999, there were 446 non-registered nursing home facilities with 20,865 beds. The number of these facilities and beds has recently decreased significantly, mainly due to many non-registered facilities converting to registered social facilities or nursing homes by the year 2000, as required by the government licensure policy.

Non-Registered Long-Term Care Facilities make up the third type of institutional care and have been long established in Taiwan. They provide a wide range of services, from home-like services to skilled nursing care. The operation of non-registered long-term care facilities is not supervised by either the health or social welfare system. Although occupancy rates run at approximately 65% to 70%, increasing demand of long-term care has seen steady growth in non-registered long-term care facilities in recent years. The scale of non-registered facilities more than doubled between 1993 and 1996, from 229 facilities with 11,790 beds to 446 facilities with 20,865 beds. It should be noted that some non-registered long-term care facilities refused to participate in the facility surveys because of their illegal status. Therefore, the actual number of non-registered long-term care facilities and places may be higher than the figures presented above.

Without supervision from either the social welfare or health system, standards of operation, personnel requirements, and quality of care are major concerns to the public. However, non-registered facilities capture the market with a relatively low cost compared to their counterpart, registered nursing homes. This cost differential may explain the rapid growth of non-registered long-term care facilities and slow growth of nursing home beds.

SERVICES AND PROGRAMS
PROVIDED BY THE HEALTH CARE SYSTEM

Compared to the history of long-term care in the social welfare system, long-term care programs and services are new to the health care system in Taiwan. The first service program organized by health care agencies was a skilled nursing home care program that began only in 1995.

The health care system is gradually giving more attention to long-term care. To meet the needs of the aging population, the Department of Health launched a *Three-Year Plan for Long-Term Care* in 1998, to run to the end of June 2001. The main objectives of this plan are:

1. To help families improve their knowledge and skills in long-term care;
2. To establish effective channels to consolidate medical care and social resources;
3. To encourage the establishment of manpower and facilities to provide pluralistic long-term care institutions; and
4. To improve laws and regulations to establish criteria for assessment of the quality of long-term care (Department of Health, 1998).

The services and programs developed by the Department of Health and the National Health Insurance again cover the three types of long-term care, that is, home care, community-based long-term care, and institutional care. In detailing these services, features that distinguish these services from equivalent services in the social welfare system are noted.

Home Care and Community-Based Long-Term Care

Visiting nursing care and day care are the two most popular services in the health care system. Whereas social welfare home care services employ only minimally trained staff, home visiting nurses in the health system services are trained to maintain disabled elderly at home as long as possible. Medical and travel expenses are covered by the National Health Insurance program. To be eligible to receive skilled nursing care at home, an elder must be bedridden at least 50% of the time, have joined the National Health Insurance program, and have a referral from a physician.

There were 221 home care agencies providing home nursing at the end of 1999. The majority are hospital-based home care services, with a small number of freestanding home care agencies. The number of elderly receiving skilled nursing care was 7,000 in 1999. This figure was expected to increase to 18,000 in 2000.

Institutional Care

The institutional settings in which long-term care services are provided include chronic hospitals and nursing homes. Nursing homes are quite a new service in the health care system compared to western countries, being formally included only after the Nurses' Law was enacted in 1991.

At the end of 1999, there were 31 freestanding nursing homes and 101 hospital-based nursing homes in Taiwan, with a total of 5,655 beds. The growth of nursing homes has been relatively slow as compared to non-registered long-term care facilities, and even compared to the registered social nursing facilities. The differences in growth rates are mainly due to the higher standards of operation and construction for nursing homes, resulting in higher costs and higher charges for services. Demand is further hindered by nursing home services not yet covered by health insurance.

Notwithstanding the slow growth in recent years, the total number of nursing home beds increased markedly to 10,385 beds in mid 2000. This increase is attributed to two health care policies. First, many public hospital beds and rural small hospitals are planning to switch their acute beds to nursing home beds because of decreasing occupancy rates; this growth will thus be achieved by conversion of existing facilities rather than new development. Second, the Department of Health is encouraging hospitals to expand their nursing home services by subsidizing interest on loans for construction. More hospital-based nursing home beds are thus expected in the near future, compared with freestanding nursing homes.

THE VETERAN ADMINISTRATION

In addition to the social welfare and health care systems, the Veteran Administration plays an important role in providing long-term care services. Only veterans are eligible for the services provided by the Veteran Administration, and traditionally, veteran homes and chronic beds at veteran hospitals have been major parts of services of the VA system that provides a range of other support services to veterans.

As Table 1 shows, veteran homes are very large scale, with 14 homes providing 15,279 places. To improve quality and efficiency of care, the VA system also plans to expand or transfer current chronic beds to nursing home beds. The 390 nursing home beds in the VA system will increase to 1,310 beds in 2000.

FRAGMENTATION IN ORGANIZATION AND DELIVERY

Due to differences in organizational structures, the provision of long-term care services in Taiwan is agency-oriented rather than service-oriented. A comprehensive model of a continuum of care has not yet been established. The fragmentation of long-term services both reflects and exacerbates problems in four areas:

1. Allocation problems due to competition for limited resources;
2. System problems due to differences in regulations and eligibility;
3. Financial problems due to different funding arrangements and misallocation of resources; and
4. Philosophical problems due to different values and beliefs about long-term care.

These problems lead to competition instead of cooperation between and among different administrations. More practically, poor linkage of long-term care services makes it difficult for disabled elders and their families to choose an appropriate long-term care program in the first place. There are three major issues for further discussion.

Accessibility

Inappropriate allocation of long-term care resources raises the issue of social equality. It is possible that those persons who are more informed may have access to better or more services compared to those who are relatively less informed. In the case of Kaohsiung City, detailed further below, it appears that a certain group of elderly may repeatedly participate in the Health Examination program, attend health education programs, and access day care, while others make little use of any services.

Efficiency

Horizontal integration among the social, health, and veteran administration systems is poorly developed due to a combination of different organizational aims and missions, values, and structures. Competition for limited resources is unavoidable, and at the same time, many long-term care resources have not been used appropriately, simply because of different structures. Lack of coordination among different long-term care systems leads to service duplication and changes the appropriate complementary relationship between social and health services to an inappropriate one of substitution.

Vertical integration is also limited because the infrastructure of each system is different. As a result, the integration and coordination of long-term care services are much more difficult, especially at the local level.

Effectiveness and Quality of Care

While both social and health systems provide nursing home services, there are differences in licensing criteria, operation standards, professional requirements, and monitoring processes. Thus, two patients with the same chronic condition may end up with two different care plans and outcomes. A further factor contributing to differences in service delivery patterns is the difference in values and beliefs about long-term care held by social welfare, health care, and clinical professionals that gives rise to different philosophies of care, at times conflicting ideologies. Diverse standards of construction of long-term care facilities also cause quality problems.

LOCAL OUTCOMES UNDER NATIONAL PROGRAMS: CASE STUDY OF KAOHSIUNG CITY

The content and organization of this paper have focused on current long-term care services and programs at the national level. With the trend to localization of services, the part played by local government has an increasing impact on the design and planning of long-term care at the local level, and contributes to variations in services at the local level. A brief account of services in Kaohsiung City, the second largest city in Taiwan, illustrates some of these developments.

While the city government has fostered the development of a wide range of services through both the social and health systems, involving community groups, the outcome is as yet a thin spread of many services rather than a coordinated regional network. In an attempt to improve coordination, some pilot projects are adopting case management approaches.

Social Care Programs

In response to the preference of most elderly Taiwanese to remain at home, Kaohsiung City government has designated specific hospitals, nursing homes, and foundations to establish training programs for home services supervisors who can provide continuous support services to those elderly with limitations in activities of daily living. By the end of October 1999, 103 home services supervisors had finished training programs and 144 elders were being served at home.

A day care center is operating as a cooperative program of public and private sectors, the Kaohsiung City Government and the Jiang-Chi Foundation. The design of the day care center is intended to provide an environment in which those elderly who have mild or moderate levels of physical, mental, and social handicaps can interact. The services provided include nursing and prevention, personal care, rehabilitation, meals, recreational and educational programs, and information services. To date, 454 elders have received full day care, and 5,132 elders have used day care as a temporary alternative.

The nutritional meal program is especially designed for those elderly who live alone, and who are bed bound or disabled. It brings together the resources of charity groups, foundations, social welfare agencies, hospitals, and qualified restaurants in the community. In general, the disabled elderly can have meals at the activity center in the community, but for those who have difficulty in getting out, home delivery of meals can be arranged. A checking service is another collaborative effort, which involves 17 volunteer groups and community agencies in monitoring the elderly living alone or with low-income, and making sure they have not become ill and unable to get help.

Two initiatives focus on caregiver support. The primary objective of the respite care program is to give temporary relief to family members who provide care to their elderly at home. However, respite programs are still in an early stage in Kaohsiung City, and from May to December 1999, only 49 elders used this program. Another service that assists family caregivers is a dementia-reporting center, which develops educational programs and activities related to dementia. In particular, the center receives reports on elderly with dementia who become lost and helps family members to find them.

Actions taken in three further areas illustrate the scope for local governments to address local needs, and the diversity of services that results. First, recognizing that housing policy has a significant role in long-term care planning, Kaohsiung City government has allocated a budget to help low-income elderly build up a safe and comfortable housing environment. Second, in order to protect the elderly from abuse, abandonment, or neglect, a protective network has been established. Specific recipients for this protective program are older residents in Kaohsiung City who need immediate help or care, or those without any support in daily living. At present, 73 cases are on the list for protective services. Third, a special program developed for the elderly living alone follows an emergent case management model. It provides a set of services including checking, meal preparation, transportation, and related services. To collect comprehensive information on those elderly who live alone, community pharmacies, clinics, and activities centers are reporting sites.

Health Long-Term Care Programs

Several financial assistance programs are available to the elderly living in Kaohsiung City, with the local government supplement assistance provided through national programs. First, senior residents are eligible for financial assistance with co-payments for National Health Insurance. Low-income elderly are also eligible to claim financial help for hospitalization, and they can receive further financial support from the city government if they spent more than US$1,583 on medical care within a three-month period.

There are three main activities underway in health promotion for older people in Kaohsiung City. One program focuses on prevention, treatment, and follow-up of hypertension and diabetic patients. Working on a case management model, public health nurses are responsible for providing information, supervising compliance, and periodic follow-up of individuals with these conditions.

In recognition of the importance in prevention, free health examinations were started in 1995 and take-up has grown rapidly. The number of elderly residents participating in 1999 was 39,000, compared to the 26,500 who participated in the first year of the program, and men have consistently outnumbered women by two to one. About 40% of the older population overall have participated, almost four times the rate for Taiwan as a whole.

The third health program, a free dental program that started in July 1999, is unique to Kaohsiung City. All elderly residents of the city are eligible to receive this service. The first stage of the program is focused on the provision of complete dentures; the second and third stages will cover those needing only partial dentures. To date, 15% of the elderly have been identified for provision of complete dentures.

SOLUTIONS AND CONCLUSIONS

The government of Taiwan recognizes that deficient linkages among long-term care services derive partly from bureaucratic organizational structures and the separate social, health, and veteran systems. Several developments are underway to address these problems. The *Three-Year Plan for Long-Term Care of the Elderly* planned by the National Department of Health serves as an example. One of the objectives of this project is to establish effective channels to consolidate medical care and social resources to provide the dependent elderly and their families with necessary assistance and support at the neighborhood or community level. To this end, the Departments of Health and Internal Affairs, the top levels of the social welfare system, have organized regular inter-organizational meetings.

At the local level, the development of a "single window" approach, akin to case management, is intended to bridge the social and health systems. The so-called "single window" calls for collaboration between social and health professionals to develop care planning from both perspectives. An elder can be assessed by one social worker and one nurse to evaluate his or her need, and suggestions and recommendations are then made, based on the results of the co-assessment. The single window approach is currently being piloted under a three-year contract project, and the results and consequences will need further evaluation.

The three-year long-term care plan also aims to revise relevant laws and regulations in order to establish criteria for assessing the quality of long-term care. Critical to this area is the development of a single assessment instrument that can be used for screening, care planning, and developing the reimbursement system for long-term care. A Chinese version of the original Minimum Data Set instrument has been developed with funding from the three-year long-term care project (Chiu, 1999), with the research providing input to the development of a Minimum Data Set internationally (Fries et al., 1997). An accreditation program for long-term care facilities is also planned for the near future.

Finally, it should be noted that several plans for developing long-term care policies and programs are still in their early stages. The results of implementation may not be able to meet the objectives perfectly, but the proposed solutions and outcomes will point the way to meeting the real challenges for long-term care for Taiwan.

REFERENCES

Brody, S. J., & Masciocchi, D. (1980). Data for long-term care planning by health systems agencies. *Am J Public Health, 70*: 1194-1198.

Chiu, H. C. et al. (1996). *Impact of National Health Insurance on the Long-Term Care System–Report*. Taipei: Department of Health.

Chiu, H. C. (1999). *Application of Minimum Data Set (MDS) in Different Types of Long Term Care Facilities in Taiwan*. Seoul: Conference presentation on 8-11 June, 1999, 6th Asia/Oceania Regional Congress of Gerontology.

Council for Economic Planning and Development, Executive Yuan (2000). *Projections of the Population of Taiwan Area, Republic of China*. Taipei: Executive Yuan.

Department of Health, Executive Yuan (1998). *Three-Year Plan for the Long-Term Care of the Elderly*. Taipei: Executive Yuan.

Department of Statistics, Ministry of the Interior, Executive Yuan (1996). *Survey of Living Conditions of the Elderly in Taiwan.* Taipei: Executive Yuan.

Fries, B. E., Schroll, M., Hawes, C., Gilgen, R., Jonsson, P. V., & Park, P. (1997). Approaching cross-national comparisons of nursing home residents. *Age and Ageing, 26,* Supplement 2: 13-18.

Lessons Learned, Questions Raised

Anna L. Howe, PhD

Consultant Gerontologist,
Immediate Past President, Australian Association of Gerontology

It has not been an easy task to draw together the wide range of themes addressed by the authors of the 14 articles in this volume who took on the task set at the Workshop held at the University of Hong Kong in early 2000. As noted in the Introduction, this task was to describe and make a critical assessment of policy and financing arrangements and service delivery in long-term care, in seven countries around the Asia-Pacific Rim. While the pairs of articles on each country have followed a common framework to a substantial degree, the content reported within these frameworks shows the enormous diversity of national long-term care systems. This diversity reflects not only the differences in the social systems and levels of economic development among the countries, but probably to an even greater degree, the diversity reflects the differences in the political, health, and welfare service structures in which the development of policies and programs takes place. That differences in these structures far outweigh similarities in demographic, social, and economic circumstances is nowhere more apparent than on either side of the United States-Canadian border.

Compared to the diversity at the macro policy level, the service delivery articles show more commonalities, and our first conclusion is that the transfer of practice concepts is easier than transfer of policy approaches. Service delivery is, then, our starting point from which to see the lessons we have learned, and we then look to questions arising in service delivery that will require policy measures for resolution. In ending with a synthesis of the questions raised for each country and across countries as long-term care systems move into the

[Haworth co-indexing entry note]: "Lessons Learned, Questions Raised." Howe, Anna L. Co-published simultaneously in *Journal of Aging & Social Policy* (The Haworth Press, Inc.) Vol. 13, No. 2/3, 2001, pp. 233-241; and: *Long-Term Care in the 21st Century: Perspectives from Around the Asia-Pacific Rim* (ed: Iris Chi, Kalyani K. Mehta, and Anna L. Howe) The Haworth Press, Inc., 2001, pp. 233-241. Single or multiple copies of this article are available for a fee from The Haworth Document Delivery Service [1-800-HAWORTH, 9:00 a.m. - 5:00 p.m. (EST). E-mail address: getinfo@haworthpressinc.com].

21st century, we see some emerging reorientations around the Pacific Rim and across the wider international scene.

PRACTICE PERSPECTIVES: LESSONS LEARNED

The evidence of transfers across service delivery systems, for example, in the adoption of standard assessment processes, the fostering of a wider range of services, and the interest in case management, points to our second conclusion which is that, notwithstanding the constraints of macro policies, practitioners have been able to bring about considerable development in delivery systems. This conclusion is especially encouraging because it shows that those involved in service delivery in long-term care are active participants in the processes of enhancing services and in advocating on behalf of those they serve. The Canadian article demonstrates the innovations that can result when local administrators and service providers are not bound by rigid programs but are able to adapt approaches from other provinces and take the initiative to develop new approaches to suit local needs. Neither is there any shortage of innovation and adaptation elsewhere, as indicated by Mehta's mention of Eldercare Cooperatives in Singapore and the local initiatives in Kaohsiung City in Taiwan, described by Chiu.

Moving from transfer on an intra-national to an international scale, Mui notes that the United States' PACE program was based on the United Kingdom's day hospital concept, and that the model has been continuously refined since it was adopted in the United States in the early 1970s. Some 30 years later, the "one door" of PACE has not only opened across the United States; it has crossed the Pacific to provide the model for Taiwan's "single window" of entry to the long-term care system.

At the same time as the accounts of service development provide many secondary lessons in how the transfer of innovative practice can be fostered, they also identify the many barriers and an inherent tension between rolling out single approaches judged to be "best practice" vis-à-vis allowing each agency itself to experiment and learn by doing. One solution noted by Mui that has potential to bridge this divide, but which has not been widely reported, is the lead agency approach in which one agency takes a leading role in supporting one or more others to adopt and adapt new practices. Such partnership offers the benefits of learning from the experience of others and promoting collaboration, but at the same time, allowing experimentation and new learning. It especially provides a mechanism for spreading the advances of demonstration and pilot projects to system-wide adoption. Our comparative perspective also alerts us to the recognition that what is "best practice" in the social and cultural context of one country may not be so appropriate in another.

The next lesson that has been learned in practice is that the set of common elements that make up an integrated service delivery system is now well established, with the broad components of assessment, provision of a mix of community care and residential care services in response to differing levels of need, and a quality assurance process. Although the delivery systems in the countries around the Pacific Rim are at different stages, there is general agreement on the kinds of services needed to support frail elderly in the community, and each country is proceeding to develop its own blend of these services. Put another way, the general recipe for long-term care services has been written and shared around, with variations coming through the addition of local flavors rather than in the basic ingredients.

With the common elements of service delivery well understood and in place to varying degrees, Rosewarne's account of the Australian system suggests that the next lesson to learn is how to bring together the separate elements of assessment, provision of care services in response to dependency, and quality assurance. Rather than seeking to refine each separate element through focusing on perfecting tools for measuring dependency and assessing care needs and then compiling various Minimum Data Sets, there may be more to be learned from making a careful selection of the tools we use, and then using them together to achieve system-wide outcomes and capture the synergistic effects of interaction among them.

PRACTICE PERSPECTIVES: QUESTIONS RAISED

It is at the system-wide level that connections between practice in service delivery and policy become critical, but before turning to the policy lessons learned, the articles on service delivery all point to the increasing professionalism of formal service delivery, and this very development poses two clear questions. The first is the compatibility between growing professionalism at the same time as a model of care centered on family care is being promoted. Taking a comparative view across the Pacific Rim countries highlights two aspects of this incompatibility. While the authors from the four Asian countries all saw changes in traditional values regarding family support for the elderly as a rationale for policies to support family caregivers, close inspection of the experience of Australia, Canada, and the United States shows that family caregiving is alive and doing reasonably well, and that it is the elderly without family who make most call on formal services. Further, and notwithstanding changes among the present younger generation, marriage and family forma-

tion have been virtually universal in the present older and middle-aged generations in the Asian countries compared to the already much larger numbers of
older people, especially older women, who have never married or remained
childless in the other countries.

These very different demographic and social patterns caution against
overgeneralization in transferring lessons about family care. Our comparative
perspective calls for a recognition that responding to these patterns will require
very different balances among approaches that (a) aim to realize latent potential for family care, whether through legislating intergenerational obligations
Singapore-style or the inclusion of cash benefits in long-term care insurance
schemes as Japan has done, (b) aim to support families in normative caregiving
roles, as in Australia's elaboration of existing programs, and (c) substitute for
the absence of families. The two former approaches aim to redefine the relative
limits of family caregiving, but the third is dealing with an absolute limit.

The capacity for family support also depends on the relative wealth of younger compared to older generations. There is no doubt that the younger generations are better off than older generations in all the Pacific Rim countries, but
there are diverging trends between the Asian countries and the others. In the
Asian countries, there is likely to be a widening gap between the older generations who had few opportunities to accumulate wealth, due in part to the lack of
retirement savings schemes, and younger generations with far greater economic
opportunities. In the other countries, the older generations have achieved a
greater level of economic security than may be possible for many in the younger
generation; the young old are the first generation to have benefited substantially
from publicly supported retirement savings schemes. The lesson to be learned is
the value of such systems for all generations.

The second and perhaps more immediate concern about professionalism is
the sustainability of systems of care that require a large professional workforce
at a time when a shortage of nurses and related care staff is emerging world-
wide. Among the several articles that recognize the need for attention to training of all levels of long-term care staff, Leung identifies the need to enhance
basic training for personal care staff in Hong Kong to complement the available
skilled workforce, and Mui identifies training of medical and allied health staff
as critical to further advances in PACE. More generally, the multidisciplinary
nature of professional involvement in long-term care requires the transfer of
learning across disciplines as well as more specialization on aged care within
particular disciplines.

Endeavors in workforce development in long-term care must be located in
the very different contexts of the United States, Canada, and Australia compared to the Asian countries. While the three former countries have all seen
enormous transformation in education and careers in the "helping professions"

in which women have traditionally been over-represented, there is a strong continuing foundation on which new training and work patterns can be built. In Hong Kong, Singapore, Japan, and Taiwan, however, the struggle to establish nursing and related occupations is occurring at a time of even greater change in women's roles and competing opportunities in other service sectors: the ground is shifting before the foundation of the long-term care workforce has even been laid.

POLICY PERSPECTIVES: COMMON CONCERNS, DIFFERING RESPONSES

Seeing that all seven countries have stated policies emphasizing community care over residential care, it would be easy to conclude that a common lesson about the balance of care had been learned. But this conclusion is quickly qualified when it is recognized that the starting point from which the balance between community and residential care is to be established is very different in each country. The Asian countries, with relatively low provision of residential care, and especially nursing home care, are now in a very different position compared to Australia, Canada, and the United States, where the goal has been to contain past growth rates. Many questions must then arise about the transferability of policies designed to address such different starting points. In Australia, the consistent application of strong national controls for more than 15 years has contained the level of provision of residential care, but has not generated a release of funding for redirection to community care, as demands for quality improvements have increased the cost of each residential place. In contrast, in the United States, Yee ably demonstrates how, in the absence of coherent national policy, long-term care has remained a residual system made up of the "left overs" from the health care and social care systems; nursing home care and home care have both been fed on the savings in health care, but many more clients have also had to find a seat at the table of long-term care.

While Hong Kong, Singapore, and Taiwan, and to a lesser extent, Japan, have the opportunity to control the level of residential care at lower levels to start, doing so will not of itself provide any resources for increasing community care. Other problems such as the underdevelopment of community care infrastructure have also been identified, and where solutions have been sought by opening the delivery of subsidized services to private-for-profit providers, outcomes have been ambivalent. The interest of private providers has not always materialized on the scale or with the efficiencies expected, but the good will of the existing not-for-profit sector has been undermined.

Community care has often been presented as offering a lower cost alternative to residential care, but a more diverse array of cost pressures have been identified. In Canada, much of the pressure has come from a shift in functions from health care to long-term care services without a commensurate shift in resources. In Australia, policy changes per se have lead to increased expenditures by government and by individual users of long-term care, but without guaranteeing commensurate increases in quality of care. In the United States, fears about potential costs as much as actual costs have posed a major barrier to considering policy options; while in Hong Kong, government has moved to contain future expenditures before the escalation begins. In all of these four countries, the main responses to concerns about financing have been framed in terms of how to control costs. Only in Japan and Singapore have questions been asked about how additional revenue could be generated to meet clearly projected increases in demand, and each has come up with a very different answer.

To the extent that Singapore's responses by way of compulsory savings schemes have built on the country's very particular social security and health insurance arrangements, these specific responses may be difficult to replicate elsewhere, but they provide two more general lessons: that even governments that are averse to public welfare can ensure a high level of social protection for the population, and that any approach to public funding of long-term care other than recurrent expenditure from general revenue needs to be consistent with and closely integrated with other social financing arrangements. Thus, as anticipated by Hong, the Singapore government's move to extend its savings system to provide basic cover for disability in old age through a new Eldershield has gained acceptance. In contrast, the Hong Kong government's Medisave proposal, which would have covered the cost of medical care rather than long-term care for older people, was not endorsed in public consultations. The difference in these outcomes can be attributed in part to the ease of extending the long-established savings approach in Singapore compared to the recent and limited take-up of social insurance schemes in Hong Kong. The Hong Kong government is now turning to integrate existing funding of medical, health, and social services and to increase the cost effectiveness of what it regards as an adequate level of expenditure on long-term care.

It is the balance between interests in long-term care rather than the balance between modes of care that comes to the fore in Yee's analysis of financing issues in the United States. She provides many salutary lessons about the limits to consumers' capacity to exercise their interests in the face of other, better organized, and more powerful interests. The three questions she poses about the roles of government as the first or last payer, as a manager of risks or of costs, and as a regulator of quality of care have been taken up to varying degrees in other articles, but they coalesce in a much broader and more basic question about the role of government in leading policy development.

IS AGING ON THE POLICY AGENDA?

Experience around the Pacific Rim shows that whether long-term care is an issue of concern for public policy does not depend on just demographic trends or changing family values or ups and downs in public expenditures. Aging becomes an issue on the policy agenda when government takes upon itself the responsibility to develop long-term care policies and provides opportunities to engage others in the policy development process.

The country in which government has accorded long-term care the highest priority is Japan, and Lai and Watanabe's articles recount the vigorous debates on the long-term care insurance scheme that have engaged a very wide range of interests for almost a decade. The governments of Hong Kong and Singapore have sponsored extensive, if somewhat more restrained, participation. Both of these governments share a reluctance to provide health and welfare services directly, but through an indirect system of incentives and compulsion, Singapore especially has ensured that the population has at least a minimum degree of social protection. A series of federal government policy initiatives and subsequent reviews has kept long-term care on the national policy agenda in Australia for more than a decade now. The latest round in this process has seen the release of the report of the Two Year Review announced in mid 1998 to monitor the radical reforms introduced in the 1997 Aged Care Act, and while some of the initial concerns have been resolved, newly identified issues will see continuing debate (Gray, 2001). In Canada, the question now coming to the fore for provincial and national governments is the extent to which inter-provincial variations in provision of long-term care will be tolerated against the long-accepted national standards for equity of access to other health care. Although at a more exploratory stage, the government of Taiwan is also taking a leading role in sponsoring policy development and planning. The United States stands out as the exception where government not only seeks to limit its direct involvement in financing and delivery of long-term care, but also eschews a leading role in policy.

WHERE WILL WE BE LOOKING FOR LESSONS IN THE YEARS AHEAD?

The 21st century seems set to bring some reorientation in the directions to which the countries around the Pacific Rim look as their long-term care systems develop. From the mid 1980s, Singapore, Hong Kong and Japan have been keen students of policies and programs in Australia, Canada, and the United States, and some of the common features seen across countries can be attributed quite readily to these exchanges. But in the coming years, Hong Kong will have a very major part to play in developing aged care in the rest of China. Taiwan is already looking to Hong Kong and cannot but be influenced by these developments. While there are many unique features to Singapore's integrated system of financing health care, retirement, and long-term care, it shares many social and cultural attributes with Malaysia and these make for a strong basis of exchange. In something of a role reversal, it will well become Australia, Canada, and the United States to take a turn at learning from the experience of long-term care insurance in Japan.

A recent report compiled by the WHO on the five countries that have legislated the provision of long-term care benefits–Austria, Germany, The Netherlands, Israel, and Japan–presages the wider scale of changes in the positions of different countries as leaders and learners in comparative long-term care (Brodsky, Habib, & Mizrahi, 2001). The search for sustainable systems of retirement income support has occupied the OECD for many years now, and the WHO report very usefully extends this search to long-term care systems not only for the frail aged but also for those with disabilities at any age.

In asking where we might look for lessons in long-term care, we can do no better than return to the United States-Canadian border, where in 1985 Robert and Rosalie Kane asked the question "What Can the United States Learn from Canada About Care for the Elderly?" as the rider to their main title, "A Will and a Way" (Kane & Kane, 1985). On reading the pairs of articles on Canada and the United States, written some 15 years later for the present volume, a pessimist might say that while much could have been learned, little has been. However, an optimist might say that these four articles, and the others in this volume, have not only provided us with many lessons; they have also informed us about why and how change has been achieved where it has, and the barriers that have thwarted progress elsewhere. This volume shows that the countries around the Pacific Rim provide many lessons in ways of caring for the frail elderly, but that the will of government to commit itself to a leading role in policy development is the most significant factor shaping the development of national long-term care systems. The question confronting us as we move into the 21st century is not so much about the ways to finance and deliver long-term care; it is more about the will of governments and those they represent to commit themselves to policies to do so.

REFERENCES

Brodsky, J., Habib, J., & Mizrahi, I. (2001). *Long-term care laws in five developed countries: A Review.* Geneva: WHO.

Gray, L. (2001). *Two year review of the aged care reforms.* Canberra: AusInfo.

Kane, R. L., & Kane, R. A. (1985). *A will and a way: What the United States can learn from Canada about caring for the elderly.* New York: Columbia University Press.

Index

Activities of Daily Living (ADLs), 77
Adult day care
    in Canada, 61,89,90
    in Singapore, 191-192
    in Taiwan, 222,225
Aged Care Assessment Teams
    (ACATS, Australia), 105,
    120
Aged cared. *See* Long-term care
Aged populations. *See* Demographic
    trends
Aging policy
    Japanese context of, 6-12
    as priority issue, 239
Alberta Resident Classification
    System (ARCS, Canada),
    74
Assessment
    in Australia, 105,120,133-135
    in Japan, 28,30
Assessment and treatment centers, in
    Canada, 90
Assisted living residences, in
    Canada, 90-91
Australia, 1,3,237
    accreditation program for care
        facilities in, 130-132
    aging as priority policy issue, 239
    assessment for care in,
        105,120,133-135
    caregiver support groups in,
        111-113
    case management in, 109,110
    changing balance of care in,
        104-108,113-115
    cost pressures in, 238
    informal caregivers in, 111-113

organization of service delivery in,
    118-120
possible developments for
    assessment process in, 133-135
quality assurance in, 129-132
recent aged care policy directions in,
    102-103
resident classification for long-term
    care facilities in, 120-129
residential care in, 118
role of Aged Care Assessment Teams
    in, 120
roles of government in aged care
    policy in, 103-104,105
structure of aged care system in,
    102,103
targeting community care in, 108-111
types of residential care facilities and
    services, 118-119

Benefit structures, 39

Canada, 1, 3
    adult day care in, 61,89,90
    aging as priority policy issue, 239
    caregiver support groups in, 90
    case-mix-based payment systems in,
        73-75,78-80
    challenges in funding long-term care
        in, 75-79
    community-based care programs,
        89-91
    cost pressures in, 238
    diversity of long-term care systems
        in, 85

establishing unified funding
   formula in, 78-79
financing long-term care and
   regionalization in, 72-73
funding for long-term care
   facilities in, 72-75
future long-term care challenges
   for, 97-98
health expenditures in, 71-72
historical context for health policy
   in, 70-71
home-based care programs in, 89
long-term care policy in, 71
managing care in diverse settings
   in, 76-77
population-based funding in, 73
provincial responsiblites for
   long-term care in, 85-87
quality management in, 93-97
regional long-term care disparities
   in, 75-76
residential care services in, 88
roles of central and provincial
   governments for health care
   services in, 84-87
service delivery at provincial level
   in, 91-93
service delivery examples at
   provincial level, 94
systemic consequences of
   long-term care funding, 79
Canada Health Act (1984), 70-71,85
Caregiver support groups
   in Australia, 111-113
   in Canada, 90
Care Managers, Japanese, 26-27
Care Ranks, for LTCI, 25-26
Carers, support for informal
   (Australia), 111-113
Case management, 41,234
   in Australia, 109,110
   in Singapore, 193-195
Case-mix-based payment systems
   (Canada), 73-75,78-80

Central Provident Fund (CPF,
   Singapore), 170-171,174
Chan, Peter, 83-99
Chi, Iris, 1-4,137-153
Chiu, Herng-Chia, 217-231
Chronic care units and hospitals, in
   Canada, 88
Community Aged Care Packages
   (CACPs), 107-108
Community care, 238
   in Australia, 108-111
   in Hong Kong, 144,166
   in Taiwan, 221
Community Care Access Centres
   (CCACs), 77,91-92
Congregate living residences, in Canada,
   90-91
Continuing care, definition of, 87

Day care. *See* Adult day care
Delivery systems, 39
Demographic trends
   in Hong Kong, 138-140
   in Japan, 9
   in Singapore, 186
   in Taiwan, 204-205,218-219
   in United States, 54-55

Elder Care Fund (Singapore), 180
Elderly Commission (Hong Kong), 143
Established Programs Financing Act
   (1977, Canada), 85

Family caregiving, 235-236
Family care homes, in Canada, 90
Financing long-term care. *See also*
   Long-term care
   in Canada, 72-79
   in Japan, 12-17
   "pillars" approach to, 182
   in Singapore, 178-179

in Taiwan, 207-209
in United States, 238-239
Functional Independence Measure
Function Related Groups
(FIM-FRGs), 75

Golden Manpower Centres
(Singapore), 196
Golden Plan (Japan), 13
Group homes, (Canada), 90

Health care, integrating, with
long-term care, 175-178
Hirdes, John P., 69-81
Home and Community Care Program
(HACC, Australia), 102,104
assessment and, 108-109
Home care
in Canada, 89
definition of, 87
LTCI and, 30-31
in Singapore, 192-193
in Taiwan, 220,221-222
Hong, Phua Kai, 169-183
Hong Kong, 1,3,237
aging as priority policy issue, 239
community care in, 144,166
cost pressures in, 238
demand for long-term care in,
159-161
demographic profile and trends of,
138-139
development of long-term system
in, 148-152
education levels of elderly in, 141
elderly care challenges in, 147-148
elderly employment in, 141
financing arrangements for
long-term care in, 143-147
future long-term care issues in,
165-168
health care in, 142

health status of, 139
housing policies in, 140
living arrangements in, 140-141
need for long-term care in, 156-159
policy commitments for aged care,
142-143
problems in providing long-term care
in, 163-164
provision of long-term care in,
151-163
residential care in, 144-146
social profile of, 139-140
social security in, 141-142
Hostels. *See* Residential care
Howe, Anna L., 1-4,101-116,233-241

Instrumental Activities of Daily Living
(IADL), 77

Japan, 1, 3, 237. *See also* Long-term
care; Long-Term Care
Insurance (LTCI, Japan)
aging as priority policy issue, 239
assessment for care in, 28,30
attempts to reform social security in,
12-17
changing family structures and
attitudes in, 9-11
cost of medical care in, 11-12
cost pressures in, 238
demographic changes in, 9
financing social security in, 12-17
Golden Plan, 13
liberalization of long-term care in,
31-33
New Golden Plan, 13
organization of long-term care in,
22-27
pension reform in, 17-19
Plan for People with Disabilities, 15
policy context for aging policy in,
6-12